Pocket Companion for

TEXTBOOK OF

Physical
Diagnosis

*One of the essential qualities of the clinician
is interest in humanity,
for the secret in the care of the patient
is in caring for the patient.*

FRANCIS WELD PEABODY
1881–1927

Pocket Companion for

TEXTBOOK OF

Physical Diagnosis,

Third Edition

Mark H. Swartz, MD, FACP

Professor of Medicine and
Marietta and Charles C. Morchand Professor of Medical Education
Director, The Morchand Center for Clinical Competence
Mount Sinai School of Medicine
New York, New York

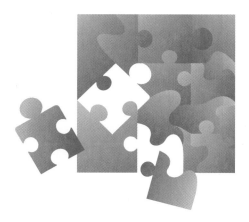

W.B. SAUNDERS COMPANY
A Division of Harcourt Brace & Company

Philadelphia London Toronto Montreal Sydney Tokyo

W.B. SAUNDERS COMPANY

A Division of Harcourt Brace & Company

The Curtis Center
Independence Square West
Philadelphia, Pennsylvania 19106

NOTICE

Medicine is an ever-changing field. Standard safety precautions must be followed, but as new research and clinical experience broaden our knowledge, changes in treatment and drug therapy become necessary or appropriate. Readers are advised to check the product information currently provided by the manufacturer of each drug to be administered to verify the recommended dose, the method and duration of administration, and contraindications. It is the responsibility of the treating physician relying on experience and knowledge of the patient to determine dosages and the best treatment for the patient. Neither the Publisher nor the author assumes any responsibility for any injury and/or damage to persons or property.

THE PUBLISHER

Library of Congress Cataloging-in-Publication Data

Swartz, Mark H.
    Pocket companion for Textbook of physical diagnosis, third edition
  / Mark H. Swartz.
        p.   cm.
    Rev. ed. of : Pocket companion to Textbook of physical diagnosis.
  c1995.
    ISBN 0–7216–7517–4
    1. Physical diagnosis—Handbooks, manuals, etc.   I. Swartz, Mark
  H.   Textbook of physical diagnosis.   II. Swartz, Mark H.   Pocket
  companion to Textbook of physical diagnosis.   III. Title.
    [DNLM: 1. Physical Examination—handbooks.   2. Medical History
  Taking—handbooks.   WB 39 S973p 1998]
  RC76.S94   1998
  616.07'5—dc21
  DNLM/DLC   97-23179

POCKET COMPANION FOR TEXTBOOK OF
PHYSICAL DIAGNOSIS, THIRD EDITION   ISBN 0-7216-7517-4

Printed in the United States of America

Last digit is the print number: 9   8   7   6   5   4   3   2   1

*To **Vivian**,*
my life's companion and best friend,
for her love, support, and understanding,

*To **Talia**,*
my wonderful and devoted daughter,

and

*To my father, **Philip**, and in memory of my mother, **Hilda**.*

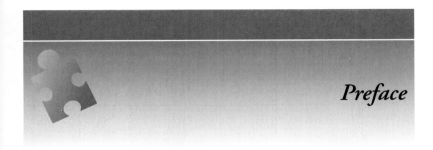

Preface

This *Pocket Companion for Textbook of Physical Diagnosis, Third Edition,* is an abbreviated, easy-to-comprehend handbook that can be conveniently carried in a coat pocket. It is more than an outline; rather it is a concise overview of the most important subjects selected from the parent textbook.

Pocket Companion for Textbook of Physical Diagnosis, Third Edition, provides a readily available pocket resource for rapid reference to subjects of interest. It should serve as a memory prompt for those studying clinical examination. The *Pocket Companion* has all the essentials of the health history and the examination steps in the evaluation of the adult patient, the pediatric patient, the pregnant patient, the geriatric patient, and the acutely ill patient. I have tried to maintain the humanistic components that are so important in the care of patients.

Although the description of each part of the history and examination is clearly stated, the pathophysiology, anatomy, impact of disease states, or detailed explanations are not discussed. When more information is required, the reader is referred to detailed coverage in the parent volume. Each topic in this pocket companion is cross-referenced with specific page numbers to their origins in the "big book."

To facilitate communication with Spanish-speaking patients, a handy chapter on useful translations has been included. An appendix listing acceptable medical abbreviations is another useful feature of this *Pocket Companion.*

It is important to emphasize that the *Pocket Companion* should not and cannot be a replacement for its parent volume, the definitive textbook. This book contains all the salient facts but is devoid of other information to enrich these facts. Also, the organization of the material is different in this volume than that in the parent volume. Thus, the two books, *Textbook of Physical Diagnosis: History and Examination,* third edition, and *Pocket Companion for Textbook of Physical Diagnosis, Third Edition,* should be considered a single educational package.

Mark H. Swartz, MD

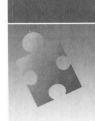

Acknowledgments

I am grateful to the endless number of patients, medical students, and faculty who have taught me medicine and a humanistic approach to patient care. To them, a quiet and respectful "thank you." I would also like to thank William Schmitt and Joan Sinclair at W.B. Saunders and Mary Espenschied for their help in putting this book together.

I have dedicated this book to my family. My wife, Vivian Hirshaut, MD, and our daughter, Talia Swartz, have tolerated the many hours of preparation and have been a constant source of strength. I am grateful to them for their efforts to review the manuscript so meticulously in order to correct my grammar and syntax. With this edition, both my wife and daughter became my best critics, editors, and proofreaders. Without their boundless affection, indefatigable help, sustained devotion, and encouragement, this book could never have come to fruition. To them, always, my deepest love.

Mark H. Swartz, MD

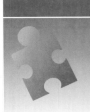

Contents

The Clinical Evaluation of an Adult Patient

CHAPTER 1

Taking a Comprehensive History from an Adult Patient

What is spoken of as a "clinical picture" is not just a photograph of a man sick in bed; it is an impressionistic painting of the patient surrounded by his home, his work, his relations, his friends, his joys, sorrows, hopes and fears.
Francis Weld Peabody
1881–1927

The main purpose of an interview is to gather all basic information pertinent to the patient's illness and the patient's adaptation to illness. An assessment of the patient's condition can then be made. An experienced interviewer considers all the aspects of the patient's presentation and then follows the leads that appear to deserve the most attention. The interviewer should also be aware of the influence of social, economic, and cultural factors in shaping the nature of the patient's problems (p. 3).

The health professional must be able to elicit and recognize a wide variety of symptoms and signs. The word *symptom* refers to what the patient feels. Symptoms are described by the patient to clarify the nature of the illness. Symptoms are *not* absolute; they are influenced by culture, intelligence, and socioeconomic background. As an example, consider the symptom of pain: patients have different thresholds of pain (p. 6).

The term *constitutional* refers to those symptoms commonly occurring with problems in any of the body systems, such as fever, chills, weight loss, or excessive sweating.

The word *sign* refers to that which the examiner finds. Signs can be observed and quantified. The major task of the interviewer is to sort out the symptoms and signs associated with a specific illness.

The diagnostic process begins at the first moment of meeting. The interviewer should greet the patient by name, make eye contact, shake hands firmly, and smile. He/she may wish to say,

- *"Mr. Smith, I'm John Jones, a medical student (or student doctor) at this hospital. I've been asked to interview and examine you."*

It is appropriate to address the patient by his or her correct title, such as Mr., Mrs., Dr., or Ms. A formal address clarifies the professional nature of the interview. Terms such as "Dear" or "Grandpa" are *not* to be used (p. 7).

If the patient is having a meal, ask if you may return when he or she is finished eating. If the patient is using a urinal or bedpan, allow privacy. Do not begin an interview in this setting. If the patient has a visitor, you may inquire whether the *patient* wishes the visitor to stay. Do not assume that the visitor is a family member. Allow the patient to introduce the person to you.

The interview can be helped or hindered by the physical setting in which the interview is conducted. If possible, the interview should take place in a quiet, well-lighted room. The curtains should be drawn around the patient's bed to create privacy. You may request that the volume of neighboring patients' radios or televisions be turned down. Lights and window shades can be adjusted to eliminate excessive glare or shade. Arrange the patient's bed light so that the patient does not feel as though under interrogation.

You should make the patient as comfortable as possible. If the patient's eyeglasses, hearing aid, or dentures were removed, ask whether he or she would like to use them. The patient may be in a chair or lying in bed. Allow the patient the choice of position. This makes patients feel that you are interested and concerned about them while it allows them some control over the interview. If the patient is in bed, it is a nice gesture to ask whether the pillows should be arranged to make him or her more comfortable.

Normally, the interviewer and the patient should be seated comfortably at the same level. To make good eye contact, the interviewer should sit in a chair directly facing the patient. The interviewer should sit in a relaxed position without crossing the arms across the chest (p. 7).

Once the introduction has been made, one may begin the interview by asking a very general, open-ended question such as, "What problem has brought you to the hospital?" This type of opening remark allows the patient to speak first. The interviewer can then determine the patient's *chief complaint*—the problem that is regarded as paramount.

When patients use terms such as "somewhat," "a little," "fair," "reasonably well," "sometimes," "rarely," or "average," the interviewer must ask for clarification. Precise communication is always desirable, and these words have been shown to have significant variations in meaning (p. 8).

The interviewer should be alert for subtle clues from the patient to guide the interview further. There are a variety of techniques to encourage and sustain the narrative. These guidelines consist of verbal and nonverbal facilitation, reflection, confrontation, interpretation, and directed questioning.

BASIC INTERVIEWING TECHNIQUES (p. 9)

Open-ended questions (e.g., *"What kind of problem are you having?"*)

Direct questions (e.g., *"Where does it hurt?"*)

Silence

Facilitation, verbal and nonverbal (e.g., *"uh, huh"* or nodding.)

Confrontation (e.g., *"You look upset."*)

Interpretation (e.g., *"You seem to be quite happy about that."*)

Reflection (e.g., *"Haven't worked since 1990?"*)

Reassurance (e.g., *"You're improving steadily!"*)

Empathy (e.g., *"I understand how difficult it must be for you."*)

FORMAT OF THE HISTORY (p. 14)

The information obtained by the interviewer is ultimately organized into a comprehensive statement about the patient's health. The interviewer should proceed through each of these major sections in a logical sequence and direct the questions relevant to each area. The format of the history is as follows (p. 14):

Source and Reliability

The *source* is usually the patient. If the patient requires a translator, the source is the patient and the translator. If family members help in the interview, their names should be included in a single-sentence statement. The reliability of the interview should also be assessed (p. 14).

Chief Complaint

The *chief complaint* is the patient's brief statement explaining why he or she sought medical attention. It is the answer to the question, "What is the problem that brought you to the hospital?" In the written history, it is frequently a quoted statement of the patient (p. 14).

History of Present Illness

The *history of the present illness* refers to the recent changes in health that led the patient to seek medical attention at this time. It describes the information relevant to the chief complaint. It should answer the questions what, when, how, where, which, who, and why (p. 14). Describe the main symptoms in terms of **location, quality, severity, timing, setting, factors that aggravate or relieve them,** and any other **associated manifestations.** The impact on the patient's life should also be indicated.

Past Medical History

The *past medical history* constitutes the overall assessment of the patient's health before the present illness. It includes all of the following:

General State of Health

As an introduction to the past medical history, the interviewer may ask, *"How has your health been in the past?"* (p. 15).

Past Illnesses

The record of *past illnesses* should include a statement of any medical, surgical, or psychiatric problem (p. 15).

Injuries

The patient should be asked about any prior *injuries* or accidents. It is important to record the type of injury and the date (p. 15).

Hospitalizations

All *hospitalizations* must be indicated. These include admissions for both medical and psychiatric illnesses (p. 15).

Surgery

All *surgical procedures* should be specified. The type of procedure, date, hospital, and surgeon's name should be obtained if possible (p. 15).

Allergies

All *allergies* should be described. These include environmental, ingestible, or drug related. The interviewer should seek specificity and verification of the patient's allergic response (p. 15).

Immunizations

It is important to determine the *immunization history* (p. 15). Record immunizations against tetanus, pertussis, diphtheria, measles, mumps, polio, influenza, hepatitis, rubella, *Pneumococcus,* and *Haemophilus influenzae.*

Substance Abuse

A careful review of any *substance abuse* by the patient is included in the past medical history. Include the type, amount, and duration of use. Substance abuse includes cigarette smoking and use of alcohol and "street drugs" (p. 16).

A history of *alcohol consumption and dependency* should be integrated into the patient's history immediately after the interviewer inquires about less-threatening subjects such as the consumption of cigarettes (p. 16).

The interviewer must ask all patients about the use of street drugs (p. 17).

Diet

When one is questioning a patient about *diet,* it is useful to ask the patient to describe what he or she ate the day before, including all three meals plus any snacks (p. 18).

Sleep Patterns

Inquire about the patient's *sleep history* (p. 18).

Current Medications

All *current medications* should be noted. If possible, ask the patient to show you the bottles and tell you how the medications are taken (p. 18). In addition to prescription drugs, include home remedies, nonprescription medications, and vitamin and mineral supplements.

Occupational and Environmental History

The *occupational and environmental history* concerns exposure to potential disease-producing substances or environments. It is important to inquire about all occupations and the duration of each (p. 18).

Biographic Information

Include the date and place of birth, sex, race, and ethnic background.

Family History

The *family history* provides information about the health of the entire family, living and dead. Include the age and health, or age and cause of death, of parents, siblings, and children, and any family history of **congenital diseases, diabetes, tuberculosis, high blood pressure, heart disease, cancer, liver disease, renal disease, headaches, arthritis, mental illness, drug addiction, or other symptoms similar to those of the patient.** One should pay particular attention to possible genetic and environmental aspects of disease that might have implications for the patient (p. 19).

Psychosocial History

The psychosocial history includes information on the education, life experiences, and personal relationships of the patient. If relevant, include religious beliefs. What is the patient's outlook on the future (p. 20)?

Sexual, Reproductive, and Gynecologic History

Obtain a *sexual, reproductive, and , if appropriate, gynecologic history.* Include sexual orientation, function, satisfaction, problems, contraceptive methods, exposure to AIDS, and precautions taken against it.

If the patient is a woman, determine **catamenia** (age at menarche, regularity, duration of periods), **last menstrual period, number of pregnancies, number of deliveries, number of abortions (or pregnancy terminations), complications of pregnancy,** and **number of living children** (pp. 21–22, 428).

Any history of *sexual, psychologic, or physical abuse* (p. 21)?

Review of Systems

The *review of systems* summarizes in terms of body systems all the many symptoms that may have been overlooked in the history of the present illness or in the past medical history. Table 1–1 is the review of systems that should be asked of all patients.

TABLE 1–1 Review of Systems

General	Current vision	Hoarseness
Usual state of health	Change in vision	Voice changes
Fever	Double vision	Postnasal drip
Chills	Excessive tearing	
Usual weight	Pain	*Neck*
Change in weight	Recent eye examinations	Lumps
Weakness	Pain when looking at light	Goiter
Fatigue	Unusual sensations	Pain on movement
Sweats	Redness	Tenderness
Heat or cold intolerance	Discharge	History of "swollen glands"
History of anemia	Infections	Thyroid trouble
Bleeding tendencies	History of glaucoma	
Blood transfusions and possible reactions	Cataracts	*Chest*
	Injuries	Cough
Exposure to radiation		Pain
	Ears	Shortness of breath
Skin	Hearing impairment	Sputum production (quantity, appearance)
Rashes	Use of hearing aid	
Itching	Discharge	Tuberculosis
Hives	"Dizziness"	Asthma
Easy bruisability	Pain	Pleurisy
History of eczema	Ringing in ears	Bronchitis
Dryness	Infections	Coughing up blood
Changes in skin color		Wheezing
Changes in hair texture	*Nose*	Last x-ray
Changes in nail texture	Nosebleeds	Last test for tuberculosis
Changes in nail appearance	Infections	History of bacille Calmette-Guérin (BCG) vaccination
History of previous skin disorders	Discharge	
	Frequency of colds	*Cardiac*
Lumps	Nasal obstruction	Chest pain
Use of hair dyes	History of injury	High blood pressure
	Sinus infections	Palpitations
Head	Hay fever	Shortness of breath with exertion
"Dizziness"		Shortness of breath when lying flat
Headaches	*Mouth and Throat*	
Pain	Condition of teeth	Sudden shortness of breath while sleeping
Fainting	Last dental appointment	
History of head injury	Condition of gums	History of heart attack
Stroke	Bleeding gums	Rheumatic fever
	Frequent sore throats	Heart murmur
Eyes	Burning of tongue	Last ECG
Use of eyeglasses		Other tests for heart function

TABLE 1–1   Review of Systems *Continued*

Vascular
Pain in legs, calves, thighs, or hips while walking
Swelling of legs
Varicose veins
Thrombophlebitis
Coolness of extremity
Loss of hair on legs
Discoloration of extremity
Ulcers

Breasts
Lumps
Discharge
Pain
Tenderness
Self-examination

Gastrointestinal
Appetite
Excessive hunger
Excessive thirst
Nausea
Swallowing
Constipation
Diarrhea
Heartburn
Vomiting
Abdominal pain
Change in stool color
Change in stool caliber
Change in stool consistency
Frequency of bowel movements
Vomiting up blood
Rectal bleeding
Black, tarry stools
Laxative or antacid use
Excessive belching
Food intolerance
Change in abdominal size
Hemorrhoids
Infections
Jaundice
Rectal pain
Previous abdominal x-rays
Hepatitis
Liver disease
Gallbladder disease

Urinary
Frequency
Urgency
Difficulty in starting the stream
Incontinence
Excessive urination
Pain on urination
Burning
Blood in urine
Infections
Stones
Bed wetting
Flank pain
Awakening at night to urinate
History of retention
Urine color
Urine odor

Male Genitalia
Lesions on penis
Discharge
Impotence
Pain
Scrotal masses
Hernias
Frequency of intercourse
Ability to enjoy sexual relations
Fertility problems
Prostate problems
History of venereal disease and treatment

Female Genitalia
Lesions on external genitalia
Itching
Discharge
Last Pap smear and result
Pain on intercourse
Frequency of intercourse
Birth control methods
Ability to enjoy sexual relations
Fertility problems
Hernias
History of veneral disease and treatment
History of diethylstilbestrol (DES) exposure
Age at menarche
Interval between periods

Duration of periods
Amount of flow
Date of last period
Bleeding between periods
Number of pregnancies
Abortions
Term deliveries
Complications of pregnancies
Description(s) of labor
Number of living children
Menstrual pain
Age at menopause
Menopausal symptoms
Postmenopausal bleeding

Musculoskeletal
Weakness
Paralysis
Muscle stiffness
Limitation of movement
Joint pain
Joint stiffness
Arthritis
Gout
Back problems
Muscle cramps
Deformities

Neurologic
Fainting
"Dizziness"
"Blackouts"
Paralysis
Strokes
"Numbness"
Tingling
Burning
Tremors
Loss of memory
Psychiatric disorders
Mood changes
Nervousness
Speech disorders
Unsteadiness of gait
General behavioral change
Loss of consciousness
Hallucinations
Disorientation

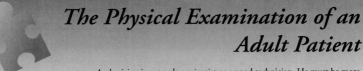

CHAPTER 2

The Physical Examination of an Adult Patient

A physician is not only a scientist or a good technician. He must be more than that—he must have good human qualities. He has to have a personal understanding and sympathy for the suffering of human beings.
Albert Einstein
1879–1955

The purpose of the chapters on physical examination is to help the student assimilate each of the individual examinations into one that is thorough and smoothly performed.

A complete examination is ideally performed in an orderly manner with as few movements required of the patient as possible. Most errors in performing a physical examination are due to a lack of organization and not to a lack of knowledge. Evaluate each part of the examination carefully before moving on to the next (p. 550).

The following examination sequence is the one that I use. There is no right or wrong sequence. Develop your own approach. Remember that at the end of whichever technique you use, the complete examination should have been performed. Whenever you change your position or that of the patient, make sure that you start "at the top" and work your way down in the examination of the body. Always remember the sequence: **inspection, palpation, percussion, and auscultation.**

In many emergency situations, the complete examination cannot and should not be performed. The health professional should, however, be familiar with all components of the examination indicated here for completeness. At the end of this chapter, an outline is provided for the assessment of the patient who is acutely ill.

In most situations, the patient will be lying in bed when you arrive. After introducing yourself and taking a complete history, you should then inform the patient that you are ready to begin the physical examination. Start by **washing your hands.**

Although it will be necessary for the patient to disrobe completely, the examination should be carried out by exposing only the areas that are being examined at that time, without undue exposure of other areas. When one is examining a woman's breasts, for example, it is necessary to check for any asymmetry by inspecting both breasts at the same time. After inspection has been completed, the physician may use the patient's gown to cover the breast not being examined. The examination of the abdomen may be done discreetly by placing a towel or the bed sheet over the genitalia. Examination of the heart with the patient in the supine position may be performed while the right breast is covered. This caring for the patient's privacy will go a long way in establishing a good doctor-patient relationship.

While performing the physical examination, the examiner should continue speaking to the patient. The examiner may wish to pursue various parts of the history, as well as telling the patient what is being done. The examiner should always refrain from comments such as "That's good" or "That's normal" or "That's fine," in reference to any part of the examination. Although such comments are initially reassuring to the patient, if the examiner fails to make such a statement during another part of the examination, the patient may automatically assume that something is wrong or abnormal.

 Patient Lying Supine in Bed

MENTAL STATUS

During the interview, the examiner has already gained much insight into the mental status of the patient. The four main components of the mental status examination are **appearance, behavior, cognition, and thought processes** (pp. 510–511).

Appearance

Assess body movements, appropriate dress, grooming, and hygiene (pp. 85–86).

Behavior

Assess Level of Consciousness (p. 511)

Is the patient awake? Alert? Is the patient's sensorium clouded by exogenous or endogenous insults? Does the patient appear confused? If necessary, touch or try to rouse the patient. If all else fails, induce pain.

Levels of Consciousness

- **Alert:** Awake or easily roused, oriented
- **Lethargic:** Somnolent, looks drowsy, often falls to sleep when not stimulated, loses train of thought
- **Delirium (acute confusional state):** Dulled cognition, impaired alertness, inattentiveness, impaired recent memory, frequently agitated, often has visual hallucinations, may be worse at night
- **Obtunded:** Sleeps most of time, is very difficult to arouse
- **Stupor (semicoma):** Responds only to vigorous shaking or induced pain, has appropriate motor responses, reflexes are present
- **Coma:** Completely unconscious, no response to pain or other stimuli, no motor activity

Evaluate mood by asking the patient about his or her mood, as well as by observing body language and facial expressions (p. 512). Note the intensity of the mood.

Assess suicide risk, if appropriate. If the patient expresses feelings of sadness, grief, or hopelessness, ask the following:

- *"Do you feel like hurting yourself?"*
- *"Have you ever had any thoughts of ending it all?"*
- *"Do you have a plan to hurt yourself?"*
- *"What would happen if you were dead?"*
- *"How would people react if you were dead?"*

Evaluate Speech (pp. 198, 511)

If the patient is awake and alert, you will have already observed the patient's speech. Note loudness, articulation, word selection, and rate and fluency of speech. The patient should now be asked to recite short phrases, such as "no ifs, ands, or buts."

Cognition

Evaluate Orientation (pp. 86, 511)

Assess the following:

- **Person:** Own name, age, type of occupation
- **Place:** Where patient lives, present location, name of city and state
- **Time:** Day of week, date, year, season

Evaluate Attention Span (pp. 512–513)

Evaluate the patient's ability to complete a thought without wandering. Is the patient distractible? Have the patient spell *W-O-R-L-D* backward. Test the patient's ability to recite *serial sevens.*

Assess Memory (pp. 512–513)

Assess *recent* memory in the context of the interview. Ask the patient to remember three words and test memory of them 5 minutes later.

Alternatively, have the patient recall as many elements in a category as possible (e.g., flowers, occupations, tools).

To test the *remote past* memory, ask the patient about well-known events in the past (e.g., birthdays, anniversaries, social security number). Don't ask about events or things that you cannot verify.

Assess Object Recognition (p. 513)

Assess Integration of Motor Activity (p. 513)

Thought Processes and Perceptions

Thought Processes

Evaluate logic, relevance, and organization of patient's thought. Does what the person says make sense?

Inquire as to any unpleasant thoughts.

Inquire about any visual or auditory perceptions.

Thought Content

Is the content consistent and logical? Inquire about any unpleasant thoughts.

Perceptions

Is the person consistently aware of reality? Inquire about any unusual perceptions (e.g., hearing or seeing things).

Judgment (p. 511)

What is the patient's insight into his or her illness? What are the patient's job plans or other plans about the future?

GENERAL APPEARANCE

1. Inspect patient's facial expression (pp. 259, 291, 366).
2. Take note of each of the following (p. 85):

- Skin color
- Apparent state of health
- Any signs of distress
- Stature and habitus
- Odors of breath or body
- Posture
- Any motor activity

Vital Signs

1. Palpate blood pressure in right arm (Fig. 2–1) (p. 296).
2. Auscultate blood pressure in right arm (Fig. 2–2) (p. 296).
3. Auscultate blood pressure in left arm (p. 298).

If blood pressure is elevated in the upper extremity, blood pressure in the lower extremity must be assessed to exclude coarctation of the aorta (p. 298).

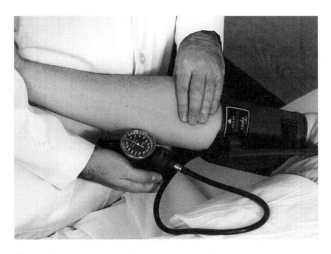

Figure 2–1   Technique for blood pressure assessment by palpation.

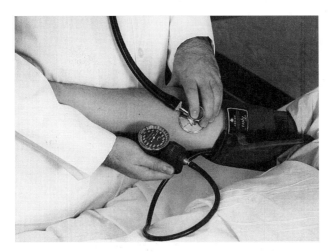

Figure 2–2   Technique for blood pressure assessment by auscultation.

 Have Patient Sit Up in Bed

Vital Signs

1. Check for orthostatic changes in the left arm (p. 297).

Have Patient Turn and Sit with Legs Dangling Off Side of Bed

Vital Signs

1. Palpate radial pulse for rate and regularity (p. 325).
2. Determine respiratory rate and pattern (p. 260).

Skin

Examine the skin for each region when the region is specifically examined (p. 98). Make note of each of the following:

1. Skin color
2. Moisture
3. Temperature
4. Texture
5. Turgor

Note any lesions present by their location, grouping, type, and color (p. 103).

Head

1. Inspect cranium for size and contour (p. 140).
2. Inspect scalp for lesions and masses (pp. 99, 140).
3. Inspect and palpate hair for quantity, distribution, and texture (p. 99).
4. Palpate cranium (p. 140).

Face

1. Inspect face for symmetry and expression (pp. 102, 140, 291, 293, 366).
2. Inspect skin on face for texture, hair distribution, and lesions (pp. 102, 140).

Eyes

1. Assess visual acuity, both eyes (p. 159).
2. Check visual fields, both eyes (Fig. 2–3) (p. 160).
3. Determine eye alignment, both eyes (p. 162).
4. Test extraocular muscle function, both eyes (Figs. 2–4 and 2–5) (p. 162).

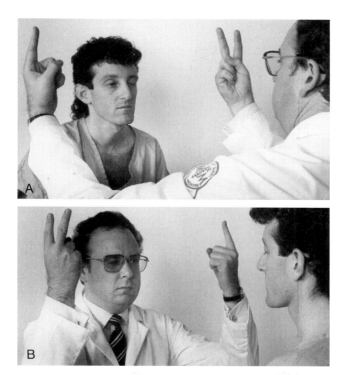

Figure 2–3   Confrontation visual field testing. *A*, View of the patient during examination of the upper fields of the right eye. *B*, Position of the examiner during examination of the upper fields of the patient's right eye.

Figure 2–4   Technique for testing ocular motility.

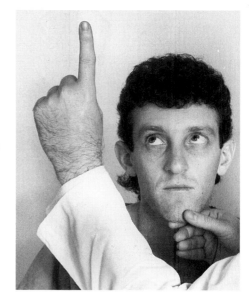

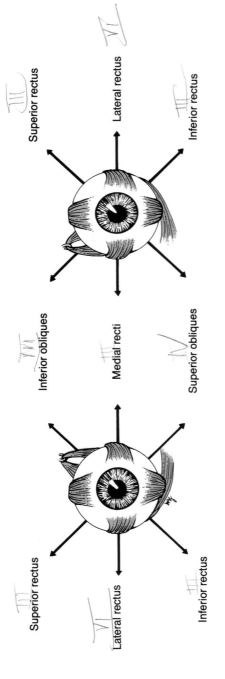

RIGHT EYE

Superior rectus

Lateral rectus

Inferior rectus

Inferior obliques

Medial recti

Superior obliques

Superior rectus

Lateral rectus

Inferior rectus

LEFT EYE

Figure 2–5   Diagnostic positions of gaze. Since the rotational actions of the obliques and vertical recti cannot be assessed, the eye must be moved into the gaze positions to maximize their vertical actions to test their innervations. The oblique muscles are tested in adduction to maximize their vertical action. The vertical recti muscles are tested in abduction, with the superior acting now as a pure elevator and the inferior as a pure depressor.

5. Check pupillary responses to light, both eyes (p. 164).
6. Inspect external eye structures, both eyes:

   - Lid (pp. 164–165, 294)
   - Conjunctiva (p. 167)
   - Sclera (pp. 167–168)
   - Cornea (p. 168)
   - Pupil—size, shape, and equality (p. 169)
   - Iris (p. 170)
   - Depth of anterior chamber (p. 170)
   - Lacrimal apparatus (p. 171)

7. Perform ophthalmoscopic examination, both eyes—arteries, veins, arteriovenous crossings, optic disc, retina, macula (Figs. 2–6 and 2–7) (pp. 172–176).

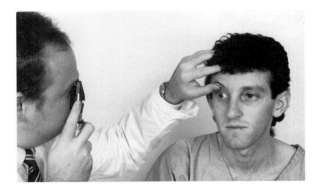

Figure 2–6   Correct position for holding the ophthalmoscope and patient's eye.

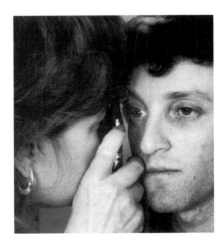

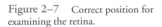

Figure 2–7   Correct position for examining the retina.

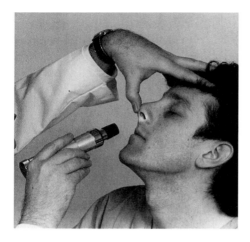

Figure 2–8   Inspection of the internal structures of the nose.

Nose

1. Inspect external portion of nose (p. 209).
2. Palpate nasal skeleton (p. 209).
3. Palpate sinuses (frontal, maxillary) for tenderness, both sides (p. 210).
4. Inspect nasal septum, both sides, noting position and integrity (Fig. 2–8) (p. 211).
5. Inspect nasal mucosa for color and swelling (p. 211).
6. Inspect turbinates, both sides (p. 211).
7. If symptoms warrant, transilluminate sinuses (p. 212).

Ears

1. Inspect external ear structures, both sides (p. 203).
2. Palpate external ear structures, both sides, noting any pain (p. 203).
3. Evaluate auditory acuity to the spoken word, both sides (pp. 203–204).
4. *If hearing is diminished,* perform Rinne test with 512 Hz tuning fork to compare air and bone conduction, both sides (Fig. 2–9) (p. 204).
5. *If hearing is diminished,* perform Weber test for lateralization with 512 Hz tuning fork (Fig. 2–10) (pp. 204–206).
6. Perform otoscopic examination, both sides (Figs. 2–11 and 2–12) (p. 206).
7. Inspect external canal, both sides (pp. 206–207).
8. Inspect tympanic membrane, both sides (pp. 207–209).

Mouth

1. Inspect outer and inner surfaces of lips, noting color (p. 229).
2. Inspect buccal mucosa, noting any sores present (Fig. 2–13) (p. 230).

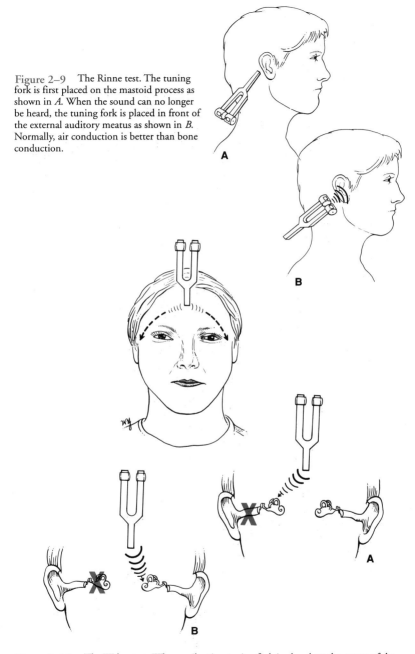

Figure 2–9   The Rinne test. The tuning fork is first placed on the mastoid process as shown in *A*. When the sound can no longer be heard, the tuning fork is placed in front of the external auditory meatus as shown in *B*. Normally, air conduction is better than bone conduction.

Figure 2–10   The Weber test. When a vibrating tuning fork is placed on the center of the forehead, the sound will be heard in the center without lateralization to either side (normal response). *A*, In the presence of a conductive hearing loss, the sound will be heard on the side of the conductive loss. *B*, In the presence of a sensorineural loss, the sound will be better heard on the opposite (unaffected) side.

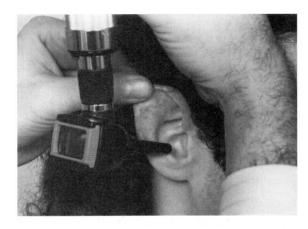

Figure 2–11   Technique for otoscopic examination. Notice that the ear is pulled up, out, and back.

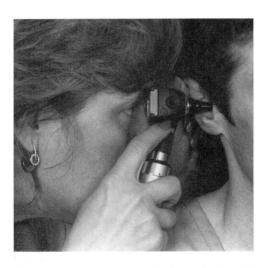

Figure 2–12   Alternative technique for otoscopic examination. The ear is again pulled up, out, and back.

3. Inspect gingivae, noting whether periodontal disease is present (pp. 231–232).
4. Inspect teeth (p. 232).
5. Inspect the tongue for papillae, symmetry, and any lesions (p. 233).
6. Palpate tongue for masses (p. 234).
7. Inspect the floor of the mouth for masses (p. 234).
8. Palpate the floor of the mouth (Fig. 2–14) (p. 235).
9. Inspect hard palate (pp. 236, 294).
10. Inspect soft palate (p. 236).
11. Observe Stensen's and Wharton's ducts, both sides (p. 234).
12. Test hypoglossal nerve function (p. 237).

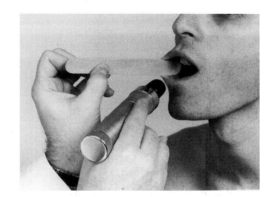

Figure 2–13   Inspection of the mouth.

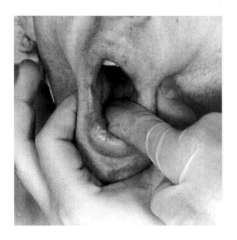

Figure 2–14   Technique for palpating oral structures.

13. Inspect the pharynx for color and exudate (p. 237).
14. Inspect the tonsils, both sides (p. 237).
15. Inspect the posterior aspect of the pharyngeal wall (p. 238).
16. Observe uvula as patient says "Ah" (p. 238).
17. Test gag reflex (p. 238).

Neck

1. Inspect neck, both sides, for masses (pp. 140, 259, 294).
2. Palpate neck, both sides, for masses (p. 140).
3. Palpate lymph nodes of head and neck, both sides (Fig. 2–15) (p. 140).
4. Palpate thyroid gland by anterior approach (Fig. 2–16) (pp. 141–142).
5. Evaluate position of trachea (pp. 267–269).
6. Evaluate mobility of trachea (Fig. 2–17) (p. 269).

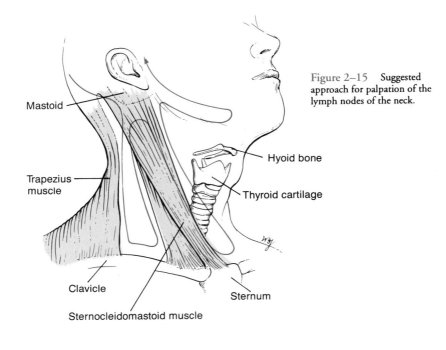

Figure 2–15 Suggested approach for palpation of the lymph nodes of the neck.

Mastoid

Trapezius muscle

Hyoid bone

Thyroid cartilage

Clavicle

Sternum

Sternocleidomastoid muscle

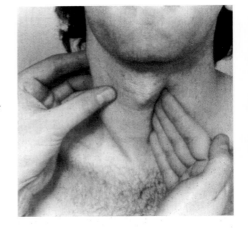

Figure 2–16 Anterior approach for palpation of the thyroid gland.

Neck Vessels

1. Inspect height of the jugular venous pulsation, right side (p. 302).

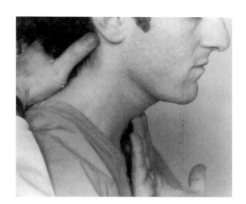

Figure 2–17 Technique for the tracheal tug.

Neck

1. Palpate thyroid gland by posterior approach* (Fig. 2–18) (p. 141).
2. Palpate for supraclavicular lymph nodes, both sides (Fig. 2–19) (p. 143).

*The examiner should now go to the back of the patient while the patient remains seated, with legs dangling off the side of the bed.

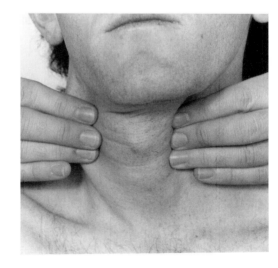

Figure 2–18 Posterior approach for palpation of the thyroid gland.

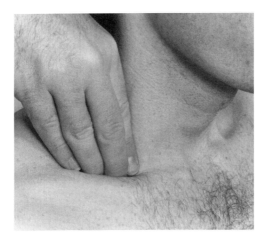

Figure 2–19 Technique for palpation of the supraclavicular lymph nodes.

Posterior Aspect of Chest

1. Inspect back for deformities, asymmetry, or masses.
2. Palpate back for tenderness, both sides (p. 262).
3. Evaluate chest excursion for symmetry, both sides (p. 262).
4. Palpate for tactile fremitus, both sides (Figs. 2–20 and 2–21) (pp. 263–264).
5. Percuss the back, both sides (Fig. 2–22) (p. 264).
6. Evaluate diaphragmatic excursion, right side (Fig. 2–23) (pp. 264–265).
7. Auscultate the back, both sides. Note the breath sounds and any adventitious sounds. Observe the quality of the sounds and their timing in the respiratory cycle (p. 267).
8. Palpate costovertebral angle for tenderness, both sides (p. 380).

Sacrum

1. Test for edema (p. 311).

Anterior Aspect of Chest*

1. Inspect patient's posture (p. 259).
2. Inspect configuration of chest (Fig. 2–24) (pp. 259–260).
3. Inspect chest, both sides.
4. Palpate for tenderness.
5. Palpate chest for tactile fremitus, both sides (p. 263).

*The examiner should now go to the front of the patient while the patient remains seated, with legs dangling off the side of the bed.

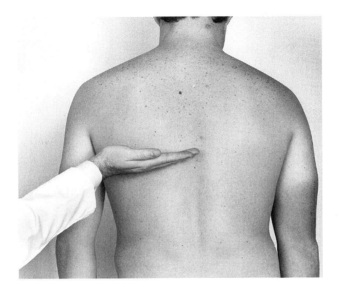

Figure 2–20   Technique for evaluating tactile fremitus.

Figure 2–21   Locations on the posterior aspect of the chest for evaluating tactile fremitus.

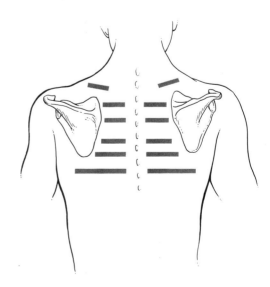

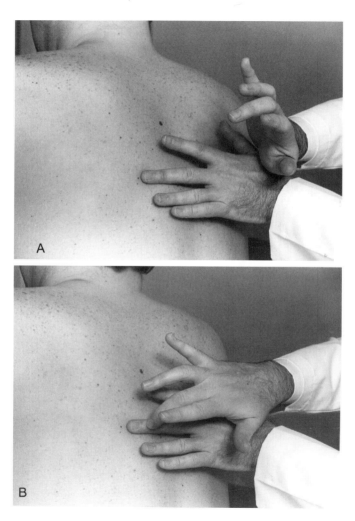

Figure 2–22   *A*, Position of the right hand ready to percuss. *B*, Location of the fingers after striking. Notice that the motion is from the wrist.

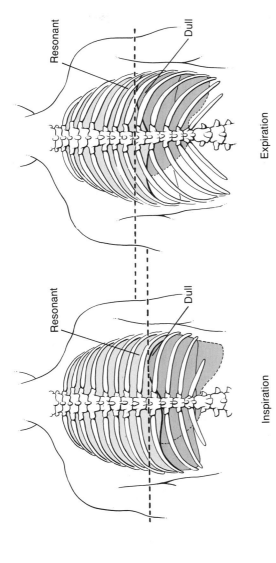

Figure 2–23 Technique for evaluating diaphragmatic motion. During inspiration, in the example on the left, percussion in the right seventh posterior interspace at the midscapular line would be resonant as a result of the presence of the underlying lung. During expiration, in the example on the right, the liver and diaphragm move up. Percussion in the same area would now be dull, owing to the presence of the underlying liver.

Inspiration

Expiration

Resonant

Dull

Resonant

Dull

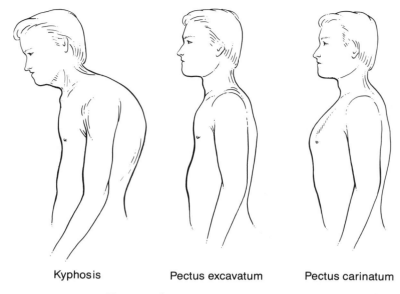

Kyphosis   Pectus excavatum   Pectus carinatum

Figure 2–24   Common chest configurations.

Female Breast

1. Inspect breasts for symmetry, size, contour, and appearance of skin, both sides (p. 344).
2. Inspect breasts for dimpling and abnormalities of contour during maneuvers to tense pectoral muscles, both sides (Fig. 2–25) (pp. 345–346).

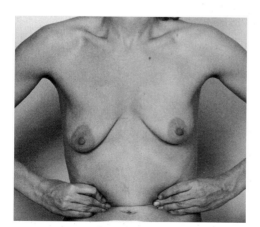

Figure 2–25   Technique for tensing the pectoralis muscles.

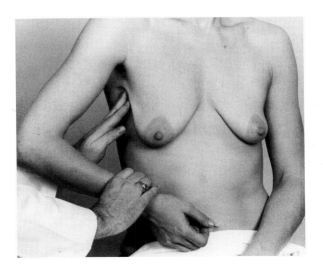

Figure 2–26   Technique for axillary examination.

Heart

1. Inspect for abnormal chest movements (p. 295).
2. Palpate for point of maximum impulse, noting location, diameter, amplitude, and duration (p. 304).
3. Auscultate for heart sounds, all four cardiac positions (pp. 306–310).

Axilla

1. Inspect axilla for rashes, infection, and pigmentation, both sides (pp. 344–345).
2. Palpate axilla for masses, both sides (Fig. 2–26) (pp. 346–347).
3. Palpate for epitrochlear nodes, both sides (p. 331).

 Have Patient Lean Forward

Heart

1. Auscultate with diaphragm at cardiac base for murmur of aortic insufficiency (Fig. 2–27) (p. 308).

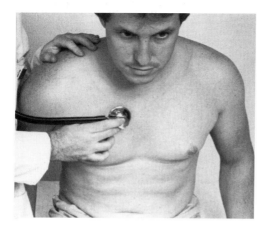

Figure 2–27   Upright, leaning-forward position for auscultation is used for listening at the base positions for aortic insufficiency.

 Have Patient Lie Supine with Head of Bed Elevated About 30 Degrees

Neck Vessels

1. Inspect the jugular venous waveform, right side (p. 300).
2. Auscultate the carotid artery, both sides (pp. 326–327).
3. Palpate the carotid artery, **each side separately,** for amplitude, contour, and any variations in amplitude or rhythm (p. 299).

Female Breast

1. Inspect breast, both sides. Note any skin changes (pp. 342, 344).
2. Palpate breast for masses, consistency, and tenderness, both sides (pp. 347–349). *If any masses are present,* note their **location, size, shape, consistency, delimitation, tenderness, and mobility** (Figs. 2–28 and 2–29).
3. Palpate subareolar area, both sides (p. 349).
4. Inspect nipple for size, shape, ulceration, or discharge.
5. Palpate nipple, both sides (Fig. 2–30) (p. 349).

Male Breast

1. Inspect the nipple and areola (p. 350).
2. Palpate the nipple, areola, and surrounding area.

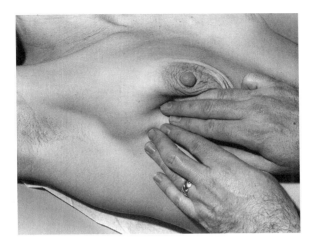

Figure 2–28   Technique for breast palpation.

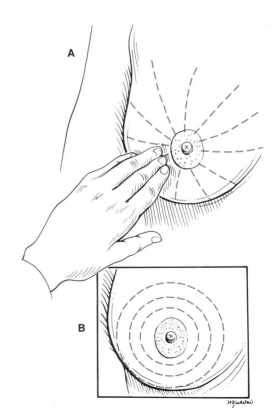

Figure 2–29   Methods of breast palpation. *A*, "Spokes of a wheel" approach. *B*, "Concentric circles" approach.

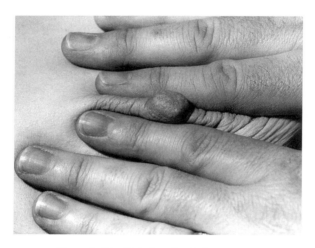

Figure 2–30   Technique for nipple examination.

Chest

1. Reinspect chest, both sides.
2. Evaluate chest excursion, both sides (p. 269).
3. Palpate for tactile fremitus, both sides (p. 269).
4. Percuss chest, both sides (Fig. 2–31) (p. 269).
5. Auscultate breath sounds, both sides (p. 270).

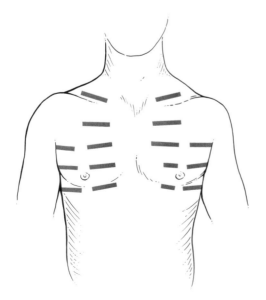

Figure 2–31   Locations on the anterior aspect of the chest for percussion.

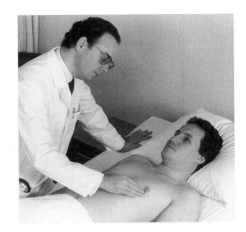

Figure 2–32 Technique for assessing localized cardiac movement.

Heart

1. Inspect for pulsations.
2. Palpate for localized motion, all four cardiac positions (Fig. 2–32) (pp. 304–305).
3. Palpate for generalized motion, all four cardiac positions (Fig. 2–33) (p. 305).
4. Palpate for thrills, all four cardiac positions (pp. 305–306).
5. Auscultate heart sounds, all four cardiac positions. Note S_1, S_2, splitting of S_2, extra systolic sounds, extra diastolic sounds, systolic murmurs, diastolic murmurs, clicks, and rubs. *If any abnormal sounds are present,* note the **time in the cardiac cycle, shape, radiation, pitch, and quality** (pp. 306–310).
6. Time the heart sounds to the carotid pulse (Fig. 2–34) (p. 308).

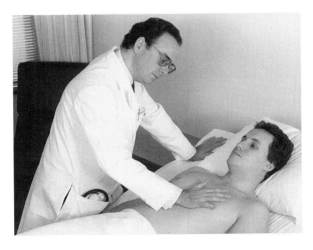

Figure 2–33 Technique for assessing generalized cardiac movement.

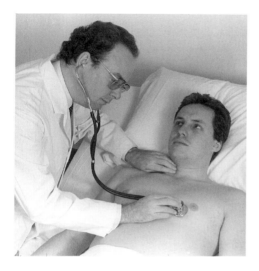

Figure 2–34   Technique for timing the heart sounds.

 Have Patient Turn on Left Side

Heart

1. Auscultate with bell at cardiac apex for murmur of mitral stenosis or S_3 (Fig. 2–35) (pp. 307–308).

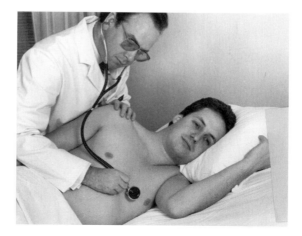

Figure 2–35   The left lateral decubitus position for auscultation is used for listening with the bell in the mitral area for mitral stenosis.

⚙ Have Patient Lie Supine with Bed Flat

Abdomen

1. Inspect the skin of the abdomen for scars and striae (Fig. 2–36) (p. 364).
2. Inspect the umbilicus and the contour of the abdomen for symmetry, enlarged organs, masses, peristaltic waves, and pulsations (pp. 366–368).

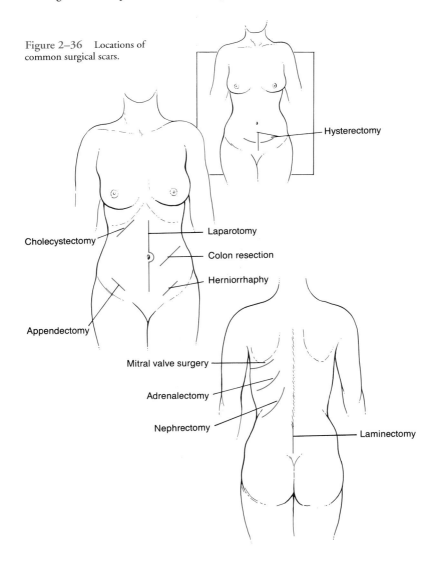

Figure 2–36   Locations of common surgical scars.

 3. Inspect for hernias (pp. 368–369).
 4. Inspect for superficial veins (p. 369).
 5. Auscultate the abdomen for bowel sounds, one quadrant (p. 370).
 6. Auscultate abdomen for bruits and friction rubs, both sides (pp. 328, 370–371).
 7. Percuss the abdomen for patterns of tympany and dullness, all four quadrants (p. 371).
 8. Percuss the right upper quadrant for span of liver dullness (Fig. 2–37) (p. 371).
 9. Percuss the left upper quadrant for splenic dullness (p. 372).
10. Test superficial abdominal reflex (p. 532).
11. Palpate abdomen lightly for guarding or tenderness, all four quadrants (p. 375).
12. Palpate abdomen deeply for masses, all four quadrants (Fig. 2–38) (p. 376).
13. *If peritoneal inflammation is suspected,* check for rebound tenderness (p. 376).
14. Check for hepatic tenderness (p. 377).
15. Evaluate the hepatojugular reflux (pp. 302–303).
16. Palpate liver for size (Fig. 2–39) (pp. 376–377). Use "hooking technique" *if necessary* (p. 377).
17. Palpate spleen for size (Fig. 2–40) (pp. 377–379).
18. Palpate kidney for enlargement (pp. 379–380).
19. Palpate aorta (p. 327).
20. Palpate for inguinal lymph nodes, both sides (p. 404).
21. *If ascites is suspected,* check for shifting dullness or a fluid wave (Figs. 2–41 and 2–42) (pp. 373–375).

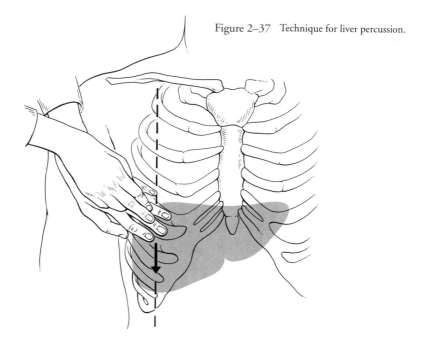

Figure 2–37   Technique for liver percussion.

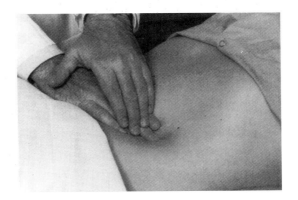

Figure 2–38   Technique for deep palpation.

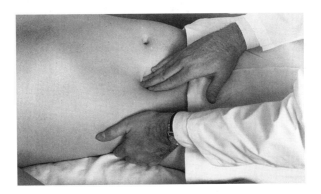

Figure 2–39   Technique for liver palpation.

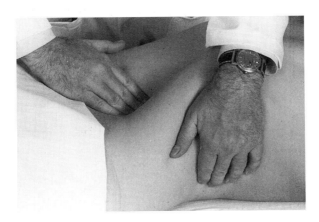

Figure 2–40   Technique for splenic palpation.

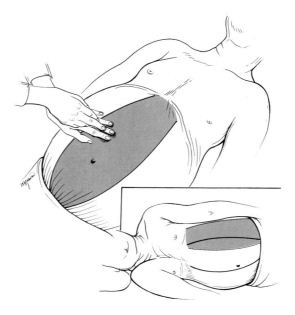

Figure 2–41   Technique for testing for shifting dullness. The colored areas represent the areas of tympany.

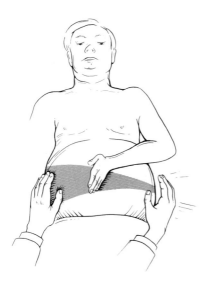

Figure 2–42   Technique for testing for a fluid wave.

Pulses

1. Palpate radial pulse, both sides (p. 325).
2. Palpate brachial pulse, both sides (pp. 325–326).
3. Palpate femoral pulse, both sides (p. 329).
4. Palpate popliteal pulse, both sides (Fig. 2–43) (pp. 329–330).
5. Palpate dorsalis pedis pulse, both sides (Fig. 2–44) (pp. 329–330).
6. Palpate posterior tibial pulse, both sides (Fig. 2–45) (pp. 329–330).
7. Time radial and femoral pulses to exclude coarctation of the aorta, right side (p. 329).
8. Perform heel-to-knee test for cerebellar disease (pp. 541–542).

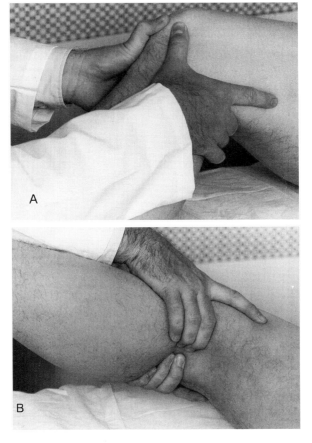

Figure 2–43 Technique for palpation of the popliteal artery. *A,* Correct position of the hands from the front. *B,* View from behind the popliteal fossa.

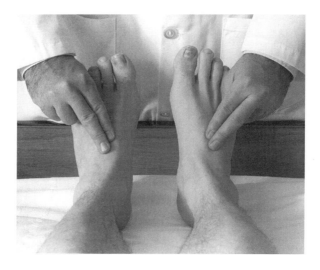

Figure 2–44 Technique for palpation of the dorsalis pedis arteries.

Legs

1. Inspect legs for size and symmetry.
2. Observe venous pattern, color and texture of skin, hair distribution.
3. Palpate for pretibial edema.

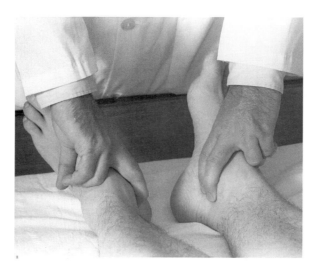

Figure 2–45 Technique for palpation of the posterior tibial arteries.

Male Genitalia

1. Inspect the skin and hair distribution to assess sexual maturity (p. 402).
2. If not already done, observe the inguinal area for masses while instructing the patient to bear down (p. 404).
3. Inspect the penis for lesions or inflammation. If man is not circumcised, retract foreskin (pp. 402, 404).
4. Inspect the scrotum for contour (p. 402).
5. Elevate the scrotum and inspect the perineum (p. 404).

 Have Man Stand in Front of Seated Examiner

Male Genitalia

1. Reinspect the penis (p. 404). Inspect the glans for signs of inflammation or lesions.
2. Inspect the external urethral meatus for location, lesions, and discharge (Fig. 2–46) (pp. 404–405).
3. Palpate the shaft of the penis for urethral stricture or masses (Fig. 2–47) (p. 406).
4. Palpate the base of the urethra (Fig. 2–48) (p. 406).
5. Reinspect the scrotum for contours. Note any rashes (pp. 403, 406).

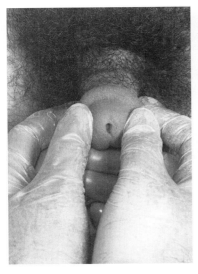

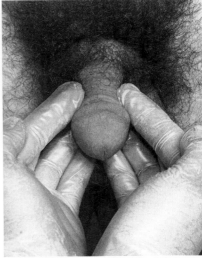

Figure 2–46 Technique for inspecting the external urethral meatus.

Figure 2–47 Technique for palpation of the penis.

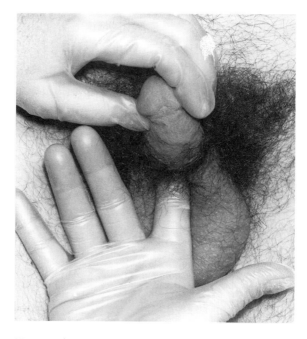

Figure 2–48   Technique for palpation of the base of the urethra.

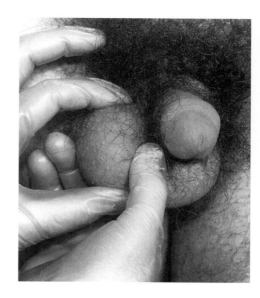

Figure 2–49   Technique for palpation of the testicle.

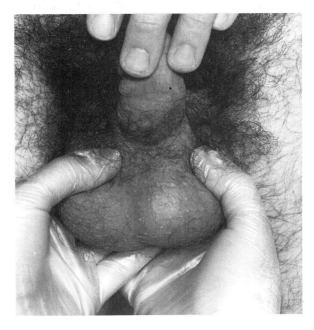

Figure 2–50   Technique for palpation of the spermatic cord.

Figure 2–51   Technique for palpation of inguinal hernias.

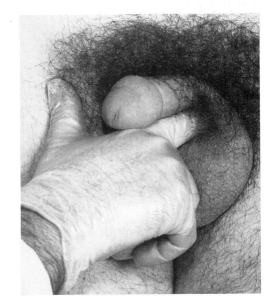

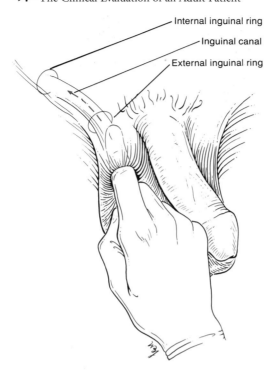

Internal inguinal ring

Inguinal canal

External inguinal ring

Figure 2–52 Position of examining finger in the inguinal canal.

6. Palpate the testicle for masses or tenderness, both sides (Fig. 2–49) (pp. 407–408).
7. Palpate the epididymis and vas deferens for tenderness, both sides (Fig. 2–50) (p. 408).
8. Inspect the inguinal area while instructing the patient to bear down (p. 410).
9. Test superficial cremasteric reflex (pp. 532–534).
10. Transilluminate any abnormal scrotal mass (p. 409).
11. Palpate for inguinal hernias, both sides (Figs. 2–51 and 2–52) (pp. 410–411).

Have Man Turn Around and Bend Over Bed

Rectum

1. Inspect the sacrococcygeal area for cysts or sinuses.
2. Inspect the perianal area for hemorrhoids, warts, or other masses (p. 381).
3. Inspect the anus while patient strains (p. 381).
4. Palpate the anal sphincter (Figs. 2–53 and 2–54) (p. 382).
5. Palpate the rectal walls for masses (pp. 382–384).
6. Palpate the prostate gland for enlargement or masses (Fig. 2–55) (pp. 384–385).
7. Test stool for occult blood (p. 385).

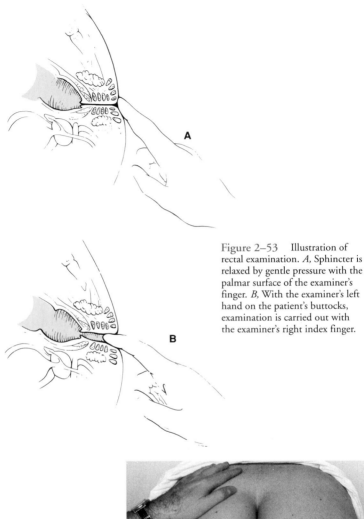

Figure 2–53   Illustration of rectal examination. *A*, Sphincter is relaxed by gentle pressure with the palmar surface of the examiner's finger. *B*, With the examiner's left hand on the patient's buttocks, examination is carried out with the examiner's right index finger.

Figure 2–54   Technique for performing rectal examination. Note position of the examiner's left hand.

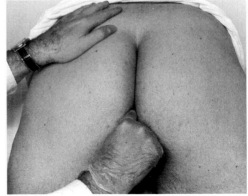

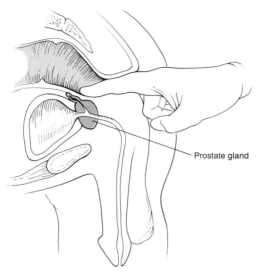

Figure 2–55   Examination of the prostate.

Prostate gland

 Woman Is Helped to Lithotomy Position

Female Genitalia

1. Inspect the skin and hair distribution to assess sexual maturity (p. 431).
2. Inspect the labia majora for inflammation, discharge, swelling, or mass lesions (p. 432).
3. Palpate the labia majora for tenderness or enlargement (p. 432).
4. Inspect the labia minora, clitoris, urethral meatus, and introitus (p. 432).
5. Inspect and palpate the area of Bartholin's glands, both sides (Fig. 2–56) (p. 432).
6. Inspect the perineum (p. 432).
7. Test for pelvic relaxation (p. 433).
8. Perform internal examination with **warmed** speculum of suitable size. Do **not** use a gel lubricant (Figs. 2–57 to 2–59) (pp. 433–434).
9. Inspect cervix for position, color, discharge, masses, or ulceration (pp. 435–436).
10. Obtain Pap smears for cytology (Fig. 2–60) (pp. 436–437).
11. Inspect vaginal walls (p. 437).
12. Perform bimanual examination to evaluate uterus and adnexa (Figs. 2–61 and 2–62) (pp. 437–438).
13. Palpate cervix and uterine body for tenderness or masses (p. 438).
14. Palpate adnexa for tenderness or masses, both sides (Fig. 2–63) (pp. 438–441).

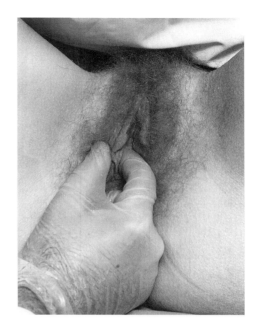

Figure 2–56 Technique for palpation of Bartholin's glands.

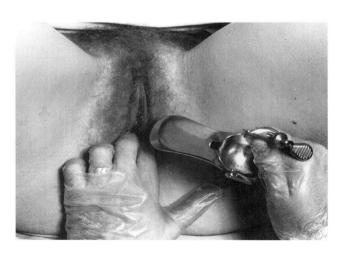

Figure 2–57 Technique for insertion of vaginal speculum. Note the examiner's fingers pressing downward on the perineum.

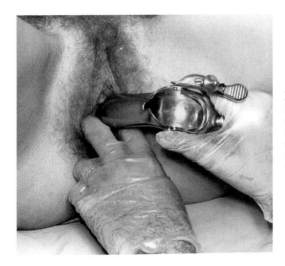

Figure 2–58 Technique for insertion of the vaginal speculum. Notice that the speculum rides over the examiner's fingers, avoiding contact with the external urethral meatus and clitoris.

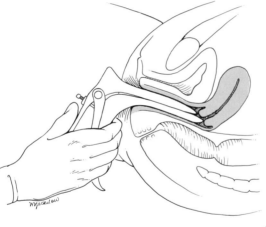

Figure 2–59 Cross-section illustrating position of the speculum during inspection of the cervix with the speculum.

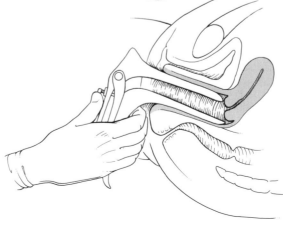

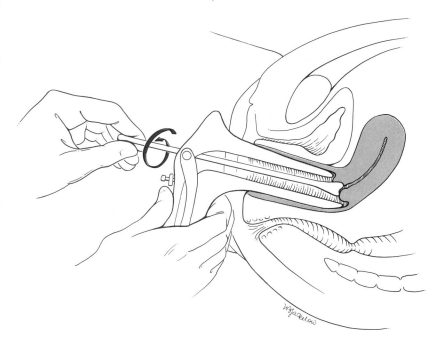

Figure 2–60 Obtaining a smear for the Pap test. Notice that the longer end of the wooden spatula is placed in the cervical os.

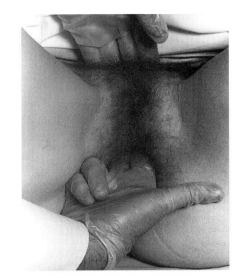

Figure 2–61 Technique for the bimanual examination.

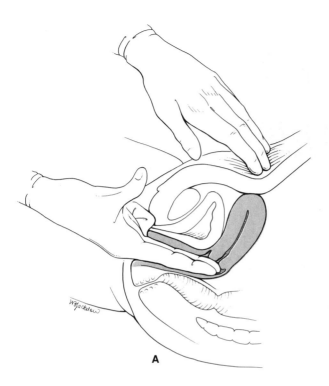

A

Figure 2–62   The bimanual examination. *A,* Cross-section through the pelvic organs. *B,* Position of the uterus between the examining hands. Notice the position of the right thumb, held away from the clitoris.

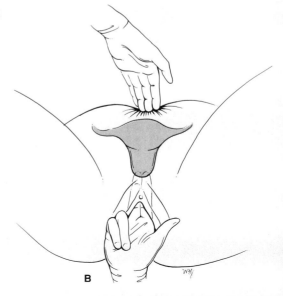

B

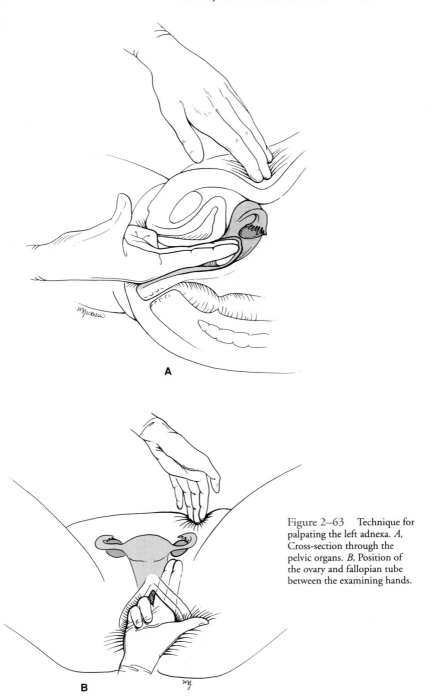

Figure 2–63 Technique for palpating the left adnexa. *A*, Cross-section through the pelvic organs. *B*, Position of the ovary and fallopian tube between the examining hands.

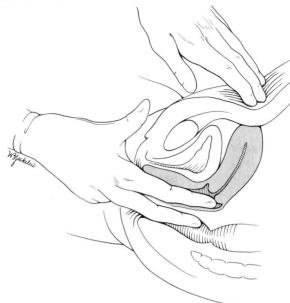

Figure 2–64   Cross-section illustrating the rectovaginal examination.

15. Palpate rectovaginal septum for thickening or masses (Fig. 2–64) (pp. 441–442).
16. Inspect and palpate anus.
17. Test stool for occult blood (p. 442).

🧩 Have Patient Sit on Bed with Legs Off Side

Face: Remainder of Neurologic and Musculoskeletal Examinations

1. Test sensory function of trigeminal nerve, both sides (Fig. 2–65) (p. 515).
2. Test motor function of trigeminal nerve, both sides (Fig. 2–66) (pp. 515–516).

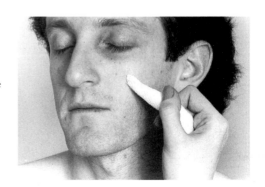

Figure 2–65   Technique for testing the sensory division of the trigeminal nerve.

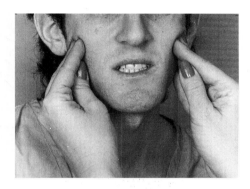

Figure 2–66 Technique for testing the motor division of the trigeminal nerve.

3. Test corneal reflex, both eyes (Fig. 2–67) (p. 515).
4. Test facial nerve, both sides (Fig. 2–68) (pp. 516–518).
5. Test spinal accessory nerve, both sides (Fig. 2–69) (pp. 519–520).
6. Test double simultaneous stimulation, both sides (Fig. 2–70) (p. 540).
7. Perform finger-to-nose test for cerebellar disease (Fig. 2–71) (p. 541).

Upper Extremities: Remainder of Neurologic and Musculoskeletal Examinations

1. Test range of motion of neck (p. 466).
2. Inspect hand and wrist, both sides (p. 472).
3. Inspect nails for color, clubbing, shape, and any lesions, both sides (pp. 99, 101, 260–261, 293).

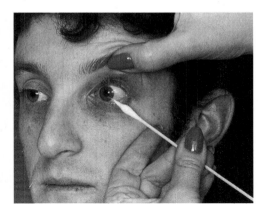

Figure 2–67 Technique for evaluating the corneal reflex.

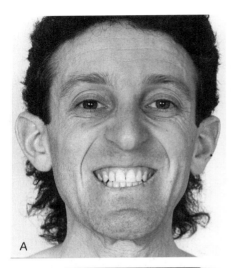

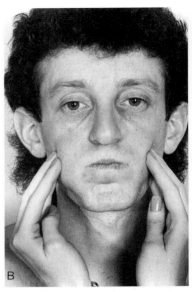

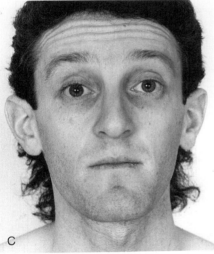

Figure 2–68   Testing the facial nerve. *A* and *B*, Tests for the lower division. *C*, Test for the upper division.

4. Palpate shoulder joint for tenderness, both sides (pp. 469–471).
5. Palpate interphalangeal joints for tenderness, both sides (p. 472).
6. Palpate metacarpophalangeal joints for tenderness, both sides (p. 472).
7. Test light touch, both sides (p. 536).
8. Test vibration sense, both sides (Fig. 2–72) (p. 538).
9. Test position sense, both sides (Fig. 2–73) (pp. 538–540).
10. Test object identification, both sides (p. 540).
11. Test graphesthesia, both sides (pp. 540–541).

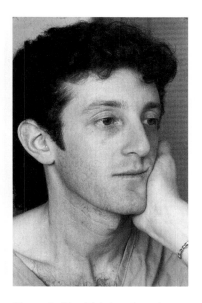

Figure 2–69   Technique for evaluating the spinal accessory nerve.

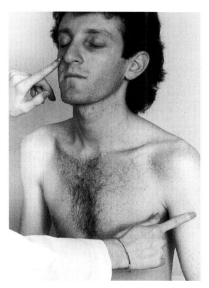

Figure 2–70   Technique for testing tactile localization.

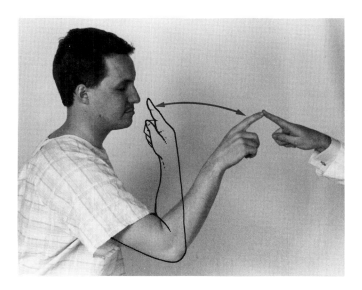

Figure 2–71   The finger-to-nose test.

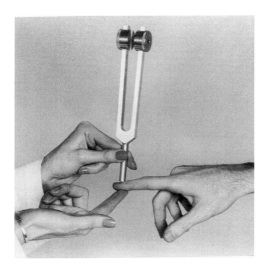

Figure 2–72 Technique for testing vibration sensation in the finger.

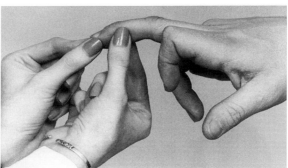

Figure 2–73 Technique for testing proprioception in the fingers.

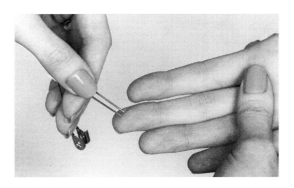

Figure 2–74 Technique for testing two-point discrimination.

12. Test two-point discrimination, both sides (Fig. 2–74) (p. 540).
13. Assess rapid alternating movements, both sides (p. 542).

Elbows: Remainder of Neurologic and Musculoskeletal Examinations

1. Inspect elbow, both sides (p. 471).
2. Test range of motion, both sides (p. 471).
3. Palpate elbow for tenderness, both sides (p. 471).
4. Test upper extremity strength, both sides (p. 468).
5. Test biceps tendon reflex, both sides (Fig. 2–75) (p. 530).
6. Test brachioradialis tendon reflex, both sides (p. 531).
7. Test triceps tendon reflex, both sides (Fig. 2–76) (p. 531).

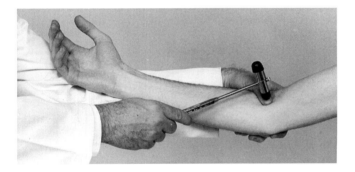

Figure 2–75   Technique for testing for the biceps tendon reflex.

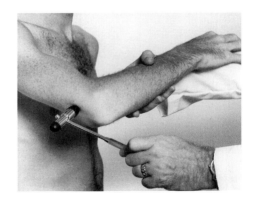

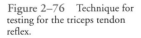

Figure 2–76   Technique for testing for the triceps tendon reflex.

Shoulders: Remainder of Neurologic and Musculoskeletal Examinations

1. Inspect shoulder, both sides (p. 469).
2. Test range of motion, both sides (p. 470).
3. Palpate shoulder joint for tenderness, both sides (p. 470).

Feet and Ankles: Remainder of Neurologic and Musculoskeletal Examinations

1. Inspect feet and ankles (p. 526).
2. Test range of motion, both sides (p. 480).
3. Palpate Achilles tendon for tenderness, both sides (p. 480).
4. Palpate metatarsophalangeal joints for tenderness, both sides (Fig. 2–77) (p. 482).
5. Palpate metatarsal heads for tenderness, both sides (p. 482).
6. Palpate ankle and foot joints for tenderness, both sides (p. 482).
7. Test light touch, both sides (p. 536).
8. Test vibration sense, both sides (Fig. 2–78) (p. 538).

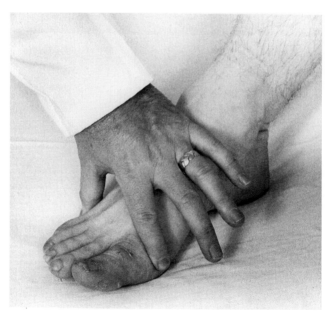

Figure 2–77   Technique for evaluating the metatarsophalangeal joints.

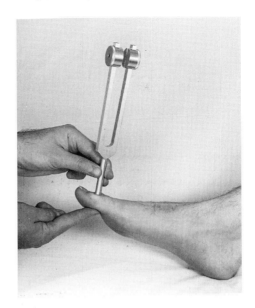

Figure 2–78   Technique for testing vibration sensation in a toe.

9. Test position sense, both sides (Fig. 2–79) (p. 538).
10. Test lower extremity strength, both sides (p. 464).
11. Test Achilles tendon reflex, both sides (Fig. 2–80) (p. 532).
12. Test plantar response, both sides (Fig. 2–81) (p. 534).

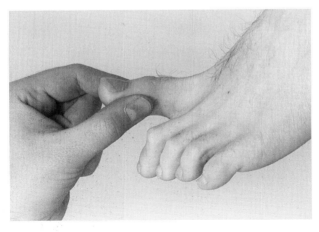

Figure 2–79   Technique for evaluating the metatarsophalangeal joints.

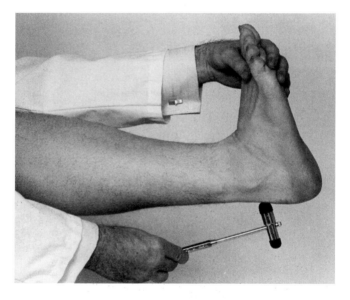

Figure 2–80   Technique for testing for the Achilles tendon reflex.

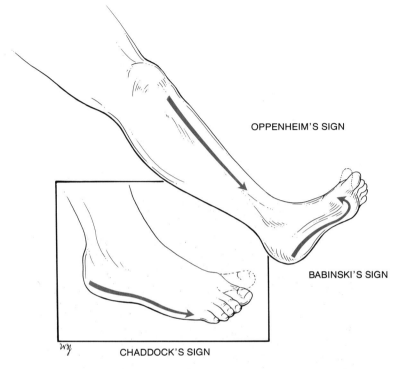

OPPENHEIM'S SIGN

BABINSKI'S SIGN

CHADDOCK'S SIGN

Figure 2–81   The plantar reflex.

Knees: Remainder of Neurologic and Musculoskeletal Examinations

1. Inspect knee, both sides (pp. 477–480).
2. Test range of motion, both sides (pp. 476–477).
3. Palpate patella for tenderness or swelling, both sides (p. 477).
4. Perform ballottement of patella if effusion is suspected (Fig. 2–82) (pp. 477–478).
5. Test patellar tendon reflex, both sides (Fig. 2–83) (p. 532).

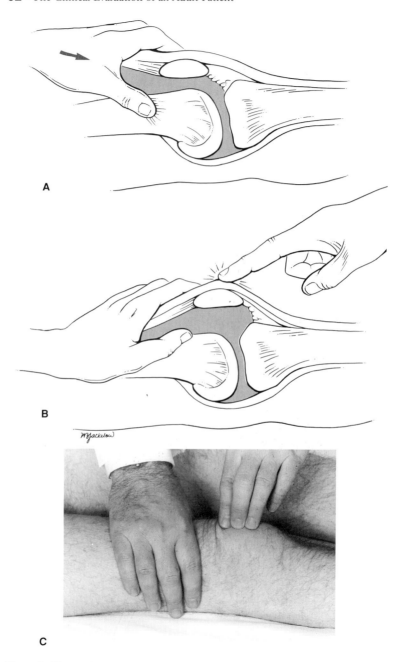

Figure 2–82   Technique for testing for a knee joint effusion. *A,* Position of the hand for pushing fluid out of the bursae. *B* and *C,* Position for tapping the patella.

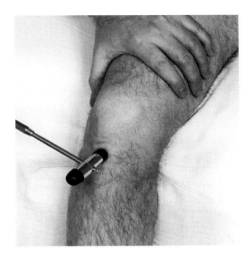

Figure 2–83   Technique for testing for the patellar tendon reflex.

 Have Patient Stand with Back to Examiner

Hips: Remainder of Neurologic and Musculoskeletal Examinations

1. Inspect hips (pp. 475–476, 526).
2. Test range of motion (p. 526).

Spine: Remainder of Neurologic and Musculoskeletal Examinations

1. Inspect spine (pp. 464, 473).
2. Palpate spine for tenderness (p. 473).
3. Test range of motion (p. 464).
4. Assess gait (pp. 464, 542–543).
5. Reinspect venous pattern in the legs.
6. Perform Romberg's test (p. 542).

The Clinical Evaluation of a Pediatric Patient

CHAPTER 3

Taking a Comprehensive History of a Pediatric Patient

Children are not like men nor women; they are almost as different creatures,
in many respects, as if they never were to be the one or the other; they are as
unlike as buds are unlike flowers, and almost as blossoms are unlike fruits.

Walter Savage Landor
1775–1864

The pediatric history, like the adult history, is obtained before the examination is performed. During this period, the child can get accustomed to the interviewer. Unlike the adult history, however, much of the pediatric history is taken from the parent or the guardian. If the child is old enough, it is very important to interview the child as well (p. 583).

Although most of the history is obtained from the parent or the guardian, some questions are asked of the child. There are two simple rules in asking questions of children:

1. **Don't ask too many questions too quickly.**
2. **Use simple language.**

The pediatric history consists of the following:

CHIEF COMPLAINT AND HISTORY OF THE PRESENT ILLNESS

Basically, the *chief complaint* and the *history of the present illness* are obtained in the same manner as with the adult patient.

PAST MEDICAL HISTORY

The *past medical history* section of the pediatric workup contains more detailed information about **immunizations** and the severity and complications of any of the **childhood illnesses** (p. 584) than the adult counterpart. Ask about **allergies,** especially eczema, urticaria, allergic rhinitis, and insect hypersensitivity. It is also important to determine the existence of allergies to penicillin, foods, or other substances (p. 585).

The most common problem associated with allergies to medications is the development of a **rash**. Rashes, however, are very common in children and may have occurred coincidentally at the time the medication was prescribed. Therefore the interviewer must determine whether the medication was the *cause* of the rash. It is also well known that certain viral states "sensitize" a patient to a medication. The medication may be given at other times without any problems (p. 585).

Record all **immunizations** with the dates given and any untoward reactions (pp. 584–585). If the child has had any **screening tests for inborn errors of metabolism, blood lead concentration, or vision or hearing deficits,** record same.

It is important to ask, "Does your child have difficulty in keeping up with other children?" The answer to this question may provide valuable information about the child's development from the parent's perspective.

BIRTH HISTORY

An important part of the pediatric history is the *birth history* (pp. 585–586). Inquire about **prenatal factors** such as the mother's health during the pregnancy. Did the mother take any medications while pregnant? Was there any vaginal bleeding during the pregnancy? What was the total weight gained?

Determine the **nature of the labor and delivery.** What was the **birth weight** (p. 586)?

At birth, was there need for any **resuscitation efforts?** Did **jaundice, cyanosis,** or **infections** occur (p. 586)?

GROWTH AND DEVELOPMENT

The *child's characteristics during infancy* indicate early developmental progress (p. 586). The **developmental milestones** are useful for helping determine normal patterns. These developmental milestones reflect the child's ability in four areas: gross motor, language, fine motor, and personal development.

The **Denver Development Screening Test (DDST)** was developed to detect development delays in the first 6 years of a child's life, with special emphasis on the first 2 years (Fig. 3–1). A line is drawn from top to bottom according to the age of the child. The examiner should test each of the milestones crossed by this line. Each milestone has a bar that indicates the percentage of the "standard" population that should be able to perform this task. Failure to perform an item passed by 90% of children is significant. Two failures in any of the four main areas indicate a developmental delay. It should be recognized that this test is a screening device for developmental delays; it is not an intelligence test.

The *current functioning of the child* provides insight into the present characteristics of the youngster. The child's social, motor, and language development and his or her maturation are reflected in current behavior. Ask the question, "How would you describe your child as a person?" (p. 586).

NUTRITION

Age-appropriate questions relating to *nutrition* are very important (p. 587). Ask about **feeding—breast or artificial.** Inquire about the frequency and duration of feed-

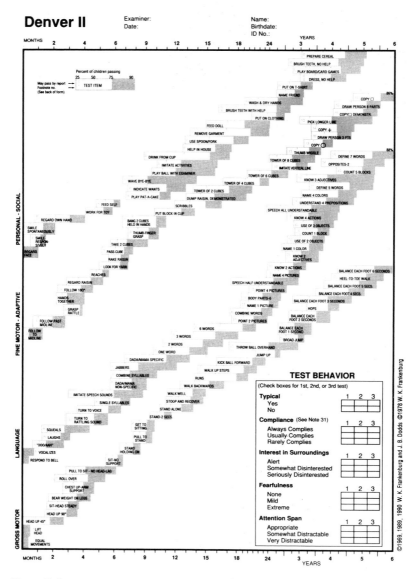

Figure 3–1   Denver Developmental Screening Test. (Reprinted with permission from William K. Frankenburg, MD, Denver Developmental Materials, Inc., Denver, Colo.)

DIRECTIONS FOR ADMINISTRATION

1. Try to get child to smile by smiling, talking or waving. Do not touch him/her.
2. Child must stare at hand several seconds.
3. Parent may help guide toothbrush and put toothpaste on brush.
4. Child does not have to be able to tie shoes or button/zip in the back.
5. Move yarn slowly in an arc from one side to the other, about 8" above child's face.
6. Pass if child grasps rattle when it is touched to the backs or tips of fingers.
7. Pass if child tries to see where yarn went. Yarn should be dropped quickly from sight from tester's hand without arm movement.
8. Child must transfer cube from hand to hand without help of body, mouth, or table.
9. Pass if child picks up raisin with any part of thumb and finger.
10. Line can vary only 30 degrees or less from tester's line.
11. Make a fist with thumb pointing upward and wiggle only the thumb. Pass if child imitates and does not move any fingers other than the thumb.

12. Pass any enclosed form. Fail continuous round motions.

13. Which line is longer? (Not bigger.) Turn paper upside down and repeat. (pass 3 of 3 or 5 of 6)

14. Pass any lines crossing near midpoint.

15. Have child copy first. If failed, demonstrate.

When giving items 12, 14, and 15, do not name the forms. Do not demonstrate 12 and 14.

16. When scoring, each pair (2 arms, 2 legs, etc.) counts as one part.
17. Place one cube in cup and shake gently near child's ear, but out of sight. Repeat for other ear.
18. Point to picture and have child name it. (No credit is given for sounds only.)
    If less than 4 pictures are named correctly, have child point to picture as each is named by tester.

19. Using doll, tell child: Show me the nose, eyes, ears, mouth, hands, feet, tummy, hair. Pass 6 of 8.
20. Using pictures, ask child: Which one flies?... says meow?... talks?... barks?... gallops? Pass 2 of 5, 4 of 5.
21. Ask child: What do you do when you are cold?... tired?... hungry? Pass 2 of 3, 3 of 3.
22. Ask child: What do you do with a cup? What is a chair used for? What is a pencil used for?
    Action words must be included in answers.
23. Pass if child correctly places and says how many blocks are on paper. (1, 5).
24. Tell child: Put block **on** table; **under** table; **in front of** me, **behind** me. Pass 4 of 4.
    (Do not help child by pointing, moving head or eyes.)
25. Ask child: What is a ball?... lake?... desk?... house?... banana?... curtain?... fence?... ceiling? Pass 5 of 8, 7 of 8.
    of use, shape, what it is made of, or general category (such as banana is fruit, not just yellow). Pass 5 of 8, 7 of 8.
26. Ask child: If a horse is big, a mouse is __? If fire is hot, ice is __? If the sun shines during the day, the moon shines during the __? Pass 2 of 3.
27. Child may use wall or rail only, not person. May not crawl.
28. Child must throw ball overhand 3 feet to within arm's reach of tester.
29. Child must perform standing broad jump over width of test sheet (8 1/2 inches).
30. Tell child to walk forward, ⊂⊃⊂⊃⊂⊃ ➤ heel within 1 inch of toe. Tester may demonstrate.
    Child must walk 4 consecutive steps.
31. In the second year, half of normal children are non-compliant.

OBSERVATIONS:

Figure 3–1 *Continued*

ing, any difficulties encountered, and the timing of weaning. Determine current eating habits (i.e., likes and dislikes, types and amounts of food eaten).

SOCIAL HISTORY

The *social history* should include the parents' occupations and the **current living conditions** and **sleeping patterns** (p. 587). It is important to determine information about **toilet training, speech problems, habitual behaviors,** and **relationships with parents, siblings, and peers.**

FAMILY HISTORY

The pediatric *family history* (p. 590) is basically the same as the adult history. It is important to obtain the names of both parents. Do not assume that a man and a woman who are with a child are the parents or that they are married. Always ask who the child's parents are. It is also important to **determine consanguinity.** The health of all siblings should be ascertained. It is important to note who the parents of all siblings are. Draw a **family tree** (p. 590).

REVIEW OF SYSTEMS

The *review of systems* is essentially the same as in the adult history (see Table 1–1). In the child's review of systems, however, there should be increased emphasis on the symptoms related to the *respiratory, gastrointestinal,* and *genitourinary* systems (p. 590).

Incest and sexual abuse are not uncommon. All children should be told that their bodies are very personal and that no one has the right to touch them or make them feel uncomfortable (p. 592). If the child is more than 3 years of age, ask the following:

• *"Has anyone touched your body in any way that made you feel uncomfortable or confused?"*

The child who has been *sexually* or *physically abused* may exhibit behavior such as **aggression, moodiness, irritability, hysteria, withdrawal, regression, memory loss, insecurity, and clinging.** In addition, the child may exhibit some of the following physical changes: **torn and/or bloody clothing, bruises or other suspicious injuries, difficulty in walking or sitting, loss of appetite, stomach problems, genital soreness or burning, difficulty in urination, vaginal or penile discharge, excessive bathing, or a desire not to bathe at all.** For the older child in school, additional problems may result, such as a drop in academic performance, prevarication, stealing, or even running away from home.

The final question in the review of systems allows the parent to discuss anything that is of concern to the parent that has not already been discussed (p. 591).

Ask the adolescent patient about the symptoms of *depression* (e.g., **body image distortion, loss of weight or appetite, lack of satisfaction, irritability, social withdrawal, drop in school performance**) (p. 591). Depression is very common, especially in girls. Ask about sexual activity, sexual abuse, and recreational drug use (p. 592). The interviewer should broach the major general areas of concern and allow the adolescent to respond.

CHAPTER 4

The Physical Examination of a Pediatric Patient

> A bodily disease, which we look upon as whole and entire within itself, may, after all, be but a symptom of some ailment in the spiritual part.
> Nathaniel Hawthorne
> 1804–1864

EXAMINATION OF THE NEWBORN INFANT

The newborn infant is assessed immediately after birth to determine the integrity of the cardiopulmonary systems. The infant is placed on a warmer, where the initial examination is conducted. Start the examination by carefully washing your hands.

The initial examination consists of evaluation of five signs *(Apgar test):*

- **Color**
- **Heart rate**
- **Reflex irritability**
- **Muscle tone**
- **Respiratory effort**

Obtain Apgar score (Table 4–1) (p. 593).

At 1 minute, a total score of 3 to 4 indicates severe cardiopulmonary depression, and the infant requires immediate resuscitative measures; a score of 5 or 6 indicates mild central nervous system depression. The tests are repeated at 5 minutes; a score equal to or greater than 8 indicates grossly normal cardiopulmonary findings.

TABLE 4–1 The Apgar Test

Sign	Score		
	0	**1**	**2**
Color	Blue, pale	Pink body with blue extremities	Completely pink
Heart rate	Absent	Below 100	Over 100
Reflex irritability*	No response	Grimace	Sneeze or cough
Muscle tone	Flaccid	Some flexion of the extremities	Good flexion of the extremities
Respiratory effort	Absent	Weak, irregular	Good crying

The acronym APGAR is useful for remembering the examinations of the Apgar test:
Appearance: color   Activity: muscle tone
Pulse: heart rate   Respiratory: respiratory effort
Grimace: reflex irritability

*This is determined by placing a soft catheter into the external nares.

General Assessment

Determine gestational age by the *Dubowitz clinical assessment* (Figs. 4–1 and 4–2 and Table 4–2) (p. 593).

The scores of the neurologic and external signs are totaled. This total is then correlated with the gestational age, according to the graph. A total score of 46 to 60 is associated

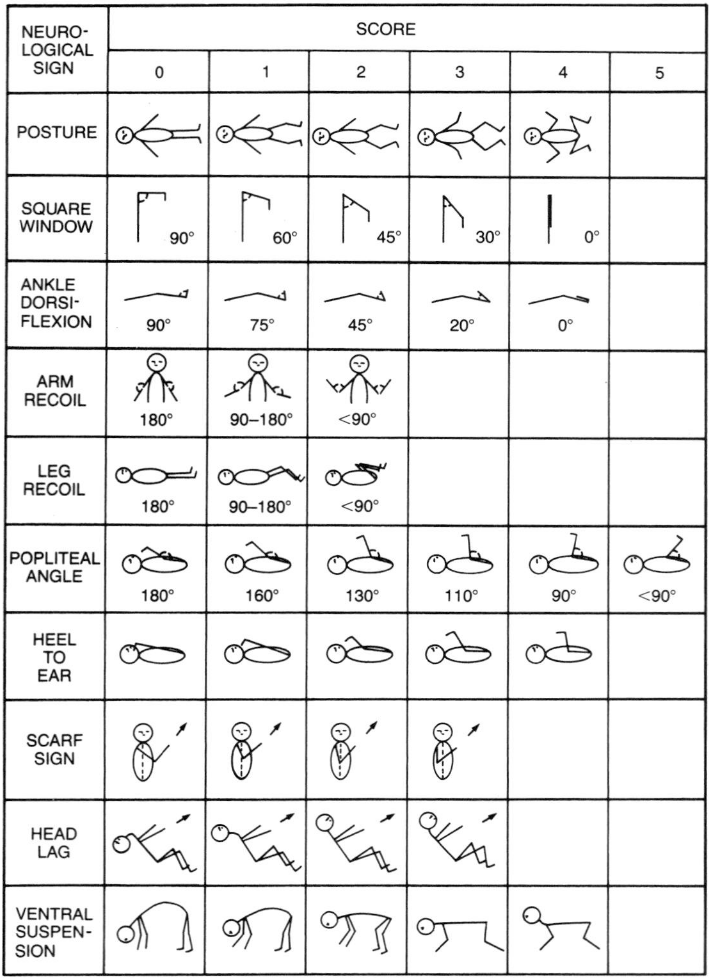

NEURO-LOGICAL SIGN	SCORE					
	0	1	2	3	4	5
POSTURE						
SQUARE WINDOW	90°	60°	45°	30°	0°	
ANKLE DORSI-FLEXION	90°	75°	45°	20°	0°	
ARM RECOIL	180°	90–180°	<90°			
LEG RECOIL	180°	90–180°	<90°			
POPLITEAL ANGLE	180°	160°	130°	110°	90°	<90°
HEEL TO EAR						
SCARF SIGN						
HEAD LAG						
VENTRAL SUSPEN-SION						

Figure 4–1   *See legend on opposite page.*

Figure 4–1   The Dubowitz Clinical Assessment. Some notes on techniques of assessment of the neurologic criteria:

Posture: Observed with infant quiet and in supine position. Score 0: Arms and legs extended; 1: beginning of flexion of hips and knees, arms extended; 2: stronger flexion of legs, arms extended; 3: arms slightly flexed, legs flexed and abducted; and 4: full flexion of arms and legs.

Square Window: The hand is flexed on the forearm between the thumb and index finger of the examiner. Enough pressure is applied to get as full a flexion as possible, and the angle between the hypothenar eminence and the ventral aspect of the forearm is measured and graded according to diagram. (Care is taken not to rotate the infant's wrist while performing this maneuver.)

Ankle Dorsiflexion: The foot is dorsiflexed onto the anterior aspect of the leg, with the examiner's thumb on the sole of the foot and other fingers behind the leg. Enough pressure is applied to get as full flexion as possible, and the angle between the dorsum of the foot and the anterior aspect of the leg is measured.

Arm Recoil: With the infant in the supine position, the forearms are first flexed for 5 seconds, then fully extended by pulling on the hands, and then released. The sign is fully positive if the arms return briskly to full flexion (score 2). If the arms return to incomplete flexion or the response is sluggish, it is graded as score 1. If they remain extended or are only followed by random movement, the score is 0.

Leg Recoil: With the infant supine, the hips and knees are fully flexed for 5 seconds, then extended by traction on the feet, and released. A maximal response is one of full flexion of the hips and knees (score 2). A partial flexion is scored 1, and minimal or no movement is scored 0.

Popliteal Angle: With the infant supine and the pelvis flat on the examining couch, the thigh is held in the knee-chest position as the examiner's left index finger and thumb support the infant's knee. The leg is then extended by gentle pressure from the examiner's right index finger behind the ankle, and the popliteal angle is measured.

Heel to Ear Maneuver: With the baby supine, draw the baby's foot as near to the head as the foot will go without forcing it. Observe the distance between the foot and the head, as well as the degree of extension at the knee. Grade according to diagram. Note that the knee is left free and may draw down alongside the abdomen.

Scarf Sign: With the baby supine, take the infant's hand and try to put it around the neck and as far posteriorly as possible around the opposite shoulder. Assist this maneuver by lifting the elbow across the body. See how far the elbow will go across and grade according to illustrations. Score 0: Elbow reaches opposite axillary line; 1: elbow between midline and opposite axillary line; 2: elbow reaches midline; and 3: elbow will not reach midline.

Head Lag: With the baby lying supine, grasp the hands (or the arms if a very small infant) and pull him or her slowly toward the sitting position. Observe the position of the head in relation to the trunk and grade accordingly. In a small infant, the head may initially be supported by one hand. Score 0: Complete lag; 1: partial head control; 2: able to maintain head in line with body; and 3: brings head anterior to body.

Ventral Suspension: The infant is suspended in the prone position, with the examiner's hand under the infant's chest (one hand in a small infant, two in a large infant). Observe the degree of extension of the back and the amount of flexion of the arms and legs. Also note the relation of the head to the trunk. Grade according to diagrams.

If score differs on the two sides, take the mean.

(Reprinted with permission from Dubowitz LMS, Dubowitz V, Goldberg C: Clinical assessment of gestational age in the newborn infant. J Pediatr 77:1-10, 1970.)

TABLE 4–2 Scoring System for External Criteria of Gestational Age

External Sign	Score*				
	0	1	2	3	4
Edema	Obvious edema of hands and feet; pitting over tibia	No obvious edema of hands and feet; pitting over tibia	No edema		
Skin texture	Very thin, gelatinous	Thin and smooth	Smooth; medium thickness. Rash or superficial peeling	Slight thickening. Superficial cracking and peeling, especially of hands and feet	Thick and parchment-like; superficial or deep cracking
Skin color	Dark red	Uniformly pink	Pale pink; variable over body	Pale; pink only over ears, lips, palms, or soles	
Skin opacity (trunk)	Numerous veins and venules clearly seen, especially over abdomen	Veins and tributaries seen	A few large vessels clearly seen over abdomen	A few large vessels seen indistinctly over abdomen	No blood vessels seen
Lanugo (over back)	No lanugo	Abundant; long and thick over whole back	Hair thinning, especially over lower back	Small amount of lanugo and bald areas	At least ½ of back devoid of lanugo

	0	1	2	3	4
Plantar creases	No skin creases	Faint red marks over anterior half of sole	Definite red marks over >anterior ½; indentations over <anterior ⅓	Indentations over >anterior ⅓	Definite deep indentations over >anterior ⅓
Nipple formation	Nipple barely visible; no areola	Nipple well defined; areola smooth and flat, diameter <0.75 cm	Areola stippled, edge not raised, diameter <0.75 cm	Areola stippled, edge raised, diameter >0.75 cm	
Breast size	No breast tissue palpable	Breast tissue on one or both sides <0.5 cm diameter	Breast tissue both sides; one or both 0.5–1.0 cm	Breast tissue both sides; one or both >1 cm	
Ear form	Pinna flat and shapeless, little or no incurving of edge	Incurving of part of edge of pinna	Partial incurving whole of upper pinna	Well-defined incurving whole of upper pinna	
Ear firmness	Pinna soft, easily folded, no recoil	Pinna soft, easily folded, slow recoil	Cartilage to edge of pinna, but soft in places, ready recoil	Pinna firm, cartilage to edge; instant recoil	
Genitals Male	Neither testical in scrotum	At least one testicle high in scrotum	At least one testicle fully descended		
Female (with hips ½ abducted)	Labia majora widely separated, labia minora protruding	Labia majora almost cover labia minora	Labia majora completely cover labia minora		

*If score differs on two sides, take the mean.

From Dubowitz LM, Dubowitz V, Goldberg C: Clinical assessment of gestational age in the newborn infant. J Pediatr 77:1–10, 1970. Adapted from Farr V, Mitchell RG, Neligan GA, et al: The definition of some external characteristics used in the assessment of gestational age in the newborn infant. Dev Med Child Neurol 8:507–511, 1966.

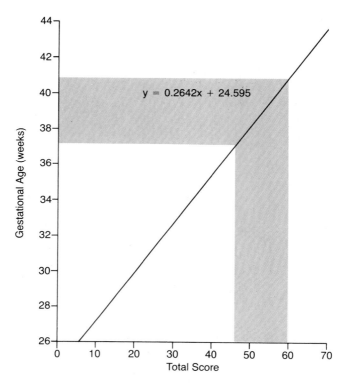

Figure 4–2   Graph for determination of gestational age based on neurologic criteria and external signs. (Reprinted with permission from Dubowitz LMS, Dubowitz V, Goldberg C: Clinical assessment of gestational age in the newborn infant. J Pediatr 77:1–10, 1970.)

with a gestational age of 37 to 41 weeks. A child with a gestational age of between 37 and 41 weeks is denoted a **term infant**. Those with gestational ages of less than 37 weeks are **preterm**; those greater than 41 weeks are **postterm**.

Weigh the newborn infant (p. 593).

Correlate the birth weight with gestational age according to the standard classification of Battaglia and Lubchenco (Fig. 4–3). Classify infant as being **small, appropriate in size, or large for gestational age** (p. 593).

The remainder of the examination is usually performed in the warmed environment of the nursery, often within 24 hours after birth.

Assess *respiratory rate* and degree of *respiratory effort* (p. 593).

Measure the *temperature* by using a rectal thermometer (p. 598).

Determine the *pulse* by auscultation of the heart (p. 598).

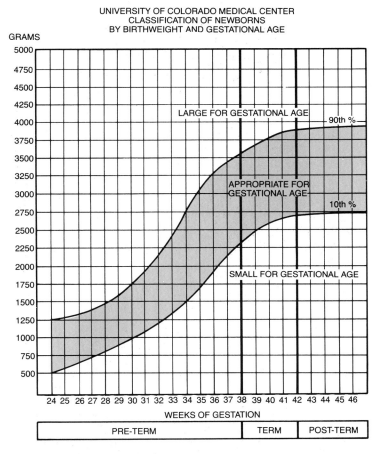

Figure 4–3   Classification of newborn infants by birth weight and gestational age. (Reprinted with permission from Battaglia FC, Lubchenco LO: A practical classification of newborn infants by weight and gestational age. J Pediatr 71:159,1967.)

Measure the head and chest (p. 598). The head is measured at its greatest circumference around the occipitofrontal area. Take three measurements and record the largest. The head circumference is usually 13.0 to 14.5 inches (34 to 37 cm). The chest circumference is normally smaller than the head circumference by 2 to 3 cm. The chest measurement is taken at the level of the nipples midway between inspiration and expiration. By the time the newborn is 1 year of age, the chest circumference will exceed the head circumference.

Measure the ratio of the upper to the lower half of the body (p. 598). The distances from the crown to the pubic symphysis and from the pubic symphysis to the heel should be compared. In the newborn infant, this ratio is 1.7:1; in the adult, the ratio is 1:1.

Measure the arm span. Normally the arm span equals the crown-to-heel length.

Although all measurements are important, the determinations of the head and chest sizes are the only routine measurements performed at this time.

Note the *posture* (p. 598).

Note the *movements* (p. 598).

Skin

Assess *skin color* (p. 598).

Inspect for *cyanosis or acrocyanosis* (p. 598).

Is *plethora* present? Is *pallor* present? Is *jaundice* present (pp. 598–599)?

Is there any evidence of *birth trauma,* manifested by petechiae, ecchymoses, or lacerations?

Observe the *pigmentation* (p. 599).

Are *vascular nevi* present (p. 599)?

Is a *rash* present (p. 600)?

Is *hair* present (p. 601)? Inspect the lumbosacral area for tufts of hair.

Examine the *dermatoglyphics* of the fingers, palms, and soles (p. 601).

Head

Assess the shape and symmetry of the *head;* assess the fontanelles (p. 601). Palpate the fontanelles.

Transilluminate the skull, if indicated (p. 602).

Inspect the *face* for symmetry (p. 602).

Eyes

Several attempts to evaluate the eyes of the newborn may be necessary. Eyelid edema related to the birth process, medications, or infection makes this part of the examination difficult.

Inspect the eyes for *symmetry* (p. 602).

Inspect the *eyelids* for evidence of trauma (p. 602).

Inspect the clarity and size of the *cornea* (p. 603).

Inspect the *iris* for clefts (p. 603).

Inspect the *conjunctivae* for hemorrhages (p. 603).

Inspect the *pupils* (p. 603).

Rotate the infant slowly to one side. The eyes should turn in the direction in which he or she is being turned. At the end of the motion, the eyes should quickly look back in the opposite direction after a few quick, nonsustained nystagmoid movements. This is termed the *rotational response.* Again place the infant on his or her back.

Assess *visual acuity* by indirect methods (p. 603).

Is the *red reflex* present? In all newborn infants, the presence of the red reflex bilaterally suggests grossly normal eyes and the absence of glaucoma or intraocular pathologic changes. Determine the presence of the red reflex by holding the ophthalmoscope 10 to 12 inches away from the eyes. The presence of the red reflex indicates that there is no serious obstruction to light between the cornea and the retina. If a red reflex is absent, *funduscopic examination* is required at this time (pp. 172–176, 603). If the red reflex is present, the examination can be postponed until the infant is 3 to 4 months of age.

Inspect the *optic disc* and the *vessels* (pp. 174, 603).

Ears

Inspect the *external ear* (p. 603). Are the ears in a normal position?

Are any *skin tags* present (p. 604)?

Test *hearing* by utilizing the primitive acoustic blink reflex (p. 604).

Inspect the *external canal.* Hold the otoscope by bracing it against the child's forehead. Insert the otoscope by pulling the pinna gently *downward* (p. 604).

Nose

Inspect for a *congenitally deviated septum.*

Assess patency of the nasopharynx by passing a soft, sterile, number 14 French catheter through each external naris and advancing it into the posterior nasopharynx (p. 604).

Mouth and Pharynx

Test the *sucking reflex.* Put on a finger cot or glove and insert your index finger into the newborn infant's mouth (p. 604).

Inspect the *gingivae.* The gums should be raised, smooth, and pink.

Inspect the *tongue.* The frenulum may be short or may extend almost to the tip of the tongue (p. 604).

Inspect the *palate.* Is there a *cleft palate?* A *bifid uvula* may be associated with a submucous cleft palate. Is the palate *high arched?* Are *petechiae* present?

Inspect for *neonatal teeth* (p. 604).

Inspect the *oropharynx* (p. 604).

Listen to the child's *cry.* Evaluate the cry for its nature, pitch, intensity, and effort (p. 604).

Neck

Is the neck *symmetric* with regard to the midline? Rotate the infant's head (pp. 604–605). Palpate for a mass in the area of the sternocleidomastoid muscle if torticollis is present.

Palpate the *clavicles* to rule out a fracture (p. 605).

Palpate for *masses* (p. 605).

Is *webbing* of the neck present (p. 605)?

Chest

Observe the *respiratory rate* while the infant is undisturbed. At several hours of age, the rate may vary from 20 to 80 breaths per minute, with an average of 30 to 40. Because of the wide variations, respirations should be counted for 1 to 2 minutes.

Inspect the *respiratory pattern.* The breathing pattern of newborn infants is almost entirely diaphragmatic. Irregular, shallow respirations are common in neonates (p. 605).

The presence of a *respiratory grunt, retractions* of the chest, or *flaring* of the nostrils indicates **respiratory distress.**

Inspect the chest for *deformities* (p. 605).

Percuss the chest by using either one finger to tap the chest or the method discussed for the adult (p. 605).

Auscultate the chest with either the bell or the small diaphragm of the stethoscope (p. 605).

Breast

Inspect the size of the breasts (p. 605). Are supernumerary nipples present along the milk line (p. 605)?

Heart

Inspect for *cyanosis* (p. 605).

Inspect for evidence of *congestive heart failure* (p. 605).

Palpate for the *point of maximum impulse* (p. 605).

Auscultate the heart in the same locations as in adults by using the small diaphragm and bell of the stethoscope (p. 606).

Pulses

Palpate the femoral pulses for a delay in the femoral pulse in comparison with the radial pulse (p. 606).

Abdomen

Inspect the abdomen for contour (p. 606).

Is an *umbilical hernia* present (p. 606)?

Inspect the *umbilical cord stump.* Is there evidence of yellow staining by meconium as a result of fetal distress (p. 606)?

Auscultate the abdomen (p. 606).

Palpate the abdomen. To relax the abdomen, use your left hand to hold the hips and knees in a flexed position while the child is sucking, and palpate with your right hand. In general, the liver edge may be felt as much as 2 cm below the right costal margin in the newborn infant (p. 606).

Palpate the *kidneys* (p. 606).

Unless clinically indicated, examination of the *rectum* is not performed (p. 606).

Genitalia

Inspect the external genitalia for *ambiguity.*

In the full-term male infant, the scrotum is relatively large and rugated. The foreskin of the penis is tight and adherent to the glans penis. Inspect the glans for the location of the external urethral meatus. The testicles should be descended into the scrotum or in the inguinal canals. Palpate the testicles by a downward movement. Are any abnormal masses present (p. 607)?

In the full-term female infant, the labia majora should cover the labia minora and clitoris. There should be a fingertip space between the vagina and the anus. Inspect the *urethral meatus* and *vaginal orifice* by placing a gloved thumb and index fingers on the child's perineum while pressing downward and laterally on the buttocks (p. 607).

Musculoskeletal Examination

The purpose of the musculoskeletal examination of a newborn is to detect gross abnormalities. The appearance of the extremities at birth usually reflects the positioning of the child within the uterus, a condition known as *intrauterine packing.*

Inspect the *extremities* and *digits.* Are all four extremities and 20 digits present?

Palpate the *clavicle* (p. 607).

Check for a *brachial palsy.*

Examine the lower extremities. Are the *hips* dislocated? Inspect the contours of the legs while the child is lying supine. The presence of asymmetric skin folds on the medial aspect of the thigh is suggestive of a proximally dislocated femur. The perineum should **not** be visible when the child is in this position, because the normal position of the thighs should cover most of it.

Place the infant's feet side by side with the soles on the examination table, allowing the hips and knees to flex. Observe the relative height of the knees. If one knee is at a lower level, you should suspect that the lower knee is the result of a dislocation of the hip on that side, a congenitally short femur, or both. If both knees are at the same height, either both hips are normal or both hips are dislocated.

Examine each hip to determine *joint stability by the Ortolani test.* Flex the neonate's legs at the hips. Hold the legs by placing your thumbs over the lesser trochanters and your index fingers over the greater trochanters, and press downward* toward the examination table. Then simultaneously abduct the hips to almost 90 degrees. The presence of a palpable or audible click suggests a dislocated hip as the femoral head

---

*This downward maneuver is known as the Barlow variation. The normal hip will not dislocate as a result of this pressure.

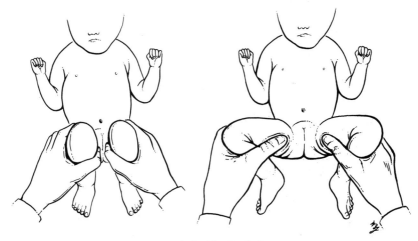

Figure 4–4   The Ortolani test.

suddenly snaps back into the acetabulum. The test should be performed *gently* on a quiet infant. **After the neonatal period, the Ortolani test result may be falsely negative** (Fig. 4–4).

Inspect the *feet*. Observe the foot at the sole (p. 608).

Neurologic Examination

Careful inspection is the most important aspect of the neonatal neurologic examination. The inspection should include the following:

- **Posture**
- **Symmetry of extremities**
- **Spontaneous movements**
- **Facial expressions and symmetry**
- **Eye movements and symmetry**

Notice the *position* of the newborn. Is hyperextension of the neck present (p. 609)?

Assess *range of motion* of all joints. Assess muscle tone and compare one side with the other. Compare the muscle sizes and strengths. Compare the resistance to passive stretch.

The *sensory* examination is generally omitted because it has low sensitivity among newborn infants.

Test the *twelfth cranial nerve* by pinching the infant's nostrils (p. 609).

Assess for *infantile automatisms* (p. 609).

Infant Lying Supine

Rooting Response

Elicited by having the infant lie with hands held against the chest. The examiner should touch the corner of the infant's mouth or cheek. The normal response is turning of the head to the same side and opening of the mouth to grasp the finger. If only the upper lip is touched, the head will retroflex; if only the lower lip is touched, the jaw will drop. The rooting response is good at 32 weeks' gestation and usually disappears after 3 to 4 months.

Plantar Grasp

Elicited by flexing the leg at the hip and knee. Dorsiflex the infant's foot with your hand. The normal response is plantar flexion of the toes over the hand. This response disappears after 9 to 12 months.

Palmar Grasp

Elicited by stabilizing the infant's head in the midline. Place your index finger into the palm of the neonate from the ulnar side. The normal response is flexion of all the fingers to grasp the index finger. If the reflex is sluggish, allow the child to suck, which normally facilitates the grasp response. The palmar grasp is usually established by 32 weeks of gestation and usually disappears after 3 to 5 months.

 Infant Picked Up and Held Supine

Moro's Reflex

Elicited by supporting the infant's body in the right hand and supporting the head in the left hand. The head is suddenly allowed to drop a few centimeters. Moro's reflex consists of symmetric abduction of the upper extremities at the shoulders and extension of the fingers. Adduction of the arm at the shoulder completes the reflex. The infant usually then emits a loud cry. Moro's reflex is one of the most important motor automatisms. The normal response indicates an intact central nervous system and is usually complete by 28 weeks of gestation. It normally disappears by 3 to 5 months of age.

 Infant Turned Over and Held Prone

Galant's Reflex

Elicited by stroking one side of infants back along a paravertebral line 2 to 3 cm from the midline from the shoulder to the buttocks. The normal response is lateral curvature of the trunk toward the stimulated side, with the shoulder and hip moving toward the side stroked. Galant's reflex normally disappears after 2 to 3 months.

Perez's Reflex

Elicited by placing your thumb at the infant's sacrum and rubbing your thumb firmly along the spine toward the infant's head. The normal response is extension of the head and spine, with flexion of the knees. Frequently the newborn infant also urinates. This reflex is normally present until 2 to 3 months of age.

 Infant Laid Down on Examination Table and Picked Up by Examiner

Placing Response; Stepping Response

Both elicited by allowing the dorsum of one of the infant's feet to touch the undersurface of a table top lightly. The normal placing response is for the infant to flex the knee and hip and place the stimulated foot on top of the table simultaneously. This response is then tested with the other foot. Placement of the soles of the feet on top of a table will elicit the stepping response, which is the alternating movements of both legs. Both these responses are best observed after 4 to 5 days of life and disappear after a period of 2 to 5 months.

EXAMINATION OF THE INFANT

Infants aged 1 week to 6 months can be examined on the examination table with a parent standing nearby. It may be easier to perform part of the examination while the infant is in the parent's arms or lap. Infants between the ages of 6 months and 1 year are best examined on the parent's lap.

Observe the infant's activity and alertness.

The more difficult portions of the examination, such as the evaluation of the pharynx and the otoscopic examination, should be performed last. Take advantage of any time when the infant is quiet to listen to the lungs and heart.

Before starting the examination, wash your hands in warm water.

General Assessment

Is any distinctive *body odor* present (p. 610)?

Evaluate pulse (p. 610).

Evaluate blood pressure by flush method, if indicated (pp. 610, 612).

Determine the infant's *length* and *weight*. Plot these measurements on the standard growth charts (Figs. 4–5 and 4–6) (p. 612).

Skin

Inspect for dermatologic conditions (p. 617).

Are any *vascular lesions* present?

Palpate the skin and assess *skin turgor* (p. 617).

Is there any evidence of physical *child abuse?* Are any bruises, welts, lacerations, or unusual scars present? Inspect the buttocks and lower back for evidence of bruises. Is there evidence of traumatic alopecia (pulling out of the hair)? Are circular, punched-out lesions of uniform size present (pp. 617–618)?

Head

Measure the *occipitofrontal* head circumference (p. 598) and chart it on the standard growth charts

Is the *face* symmetric (p. 618)?

Eyes

In an infant more than 3 weeks of age, check the *pupillary responses* (p. 618).

The production of *tears* begins at about 2 to 3 months of age, but the nasolacrimal duct is not fully patent until 5 to 7 months. If chronic tearing is present, the nasolacrimal duct may not be patent. In this case, massaging over the nasolacrimal sac may yield a purulent or mucoid discharge, which suggests the diagnosis of nasolacrimal obstruction.

Assess *visual acuity* by qualitative observations. By the age of 4 weeks, the infant should be capable of fixation on a target. By 6 weeks, coordinated eye movements in following an object should be present. At the age of 3 months, the normal infant can visually follow an object moving across the midline. Convergence is also present by this time.

Is *optokinetic nystagmus* present (pp. 618–619)?

Observe *ocular motility* in a child 3 months of age or older. Have the child follow an object into the various positions of gaze. Alignment of the eyes is best determined by the symmetry of the *corneal light reflex* and the *alternate cover test* (p. 162).

Nose

Elevate the tip of the nose to view the nasal septum, floor of the nose, and the turbinates. Are any masses or *foreign bodies* present (p. 619)?

Neck

Palpate for lymphadenopathy (p. 141).

Check for *nuchal rigidity,* if meningitis is suspected, with the Brudzinski and Kernig tests (pp. 544–547).

Chest

The examination of the chest is best performed while the infant is either sleeping or held by a parent.

Often the tracheal breath sounds are transmitted down to the chest. Be careful not to misinterpret these sounds as crackles.

Is the child in *respiratory distress?* The most important signs of distress are the use of accessory muscles, head bobbing, and flaring of the nasal alae. Intercostal retractions are also commonly present.

Percuss and auscultate the lung fields (pp. 264, 265–266).

Heart

Is *cyanosis* present (p. 619)?

Inspect for evidence of *congestive heart failure.* The most important signs are persistent tachycardia, tachypnea, and an enlarged liver. A persistent tachycardia, with a heart rate of more than 200 beats/min in newborn infants or more than 150 beats/min in children up to 1 year of age should alert the examiner (p. 619).

Palpate for the *point of maximum impulse* (p. 304).

Auscultate the heart. Heart sounds S_3 and an S_4 are very common in this age group. The clinical significance of a murmur heard, especially in the first few weeks of life, must be carefully assessed.

Abdomen

Inspect the *umbilicus.* Observe the abdomen for any masses. An umbilical hernia is not uncommon in this age group, especially in the African-American and Latino populations (p. 620). *Text continued on page 94.*

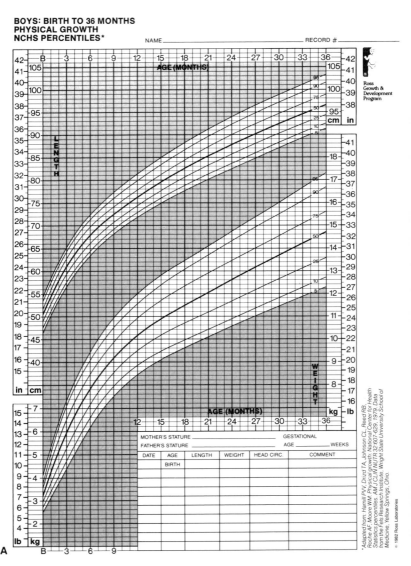

Figure 4–5A   National Center for Health Statistics (NCHS) growth charts, birth to age 36 months. *A,* The NCHS percentiles for boys. (Figures provided through the courtesy of Ross Laboratories, Columbus, Ohio.)

BOYS: BIRTH TO 36 MONTHS
PHYSICAL GROWTH
NCHS PERCENTILES*

NAME _____ RECORD # _____

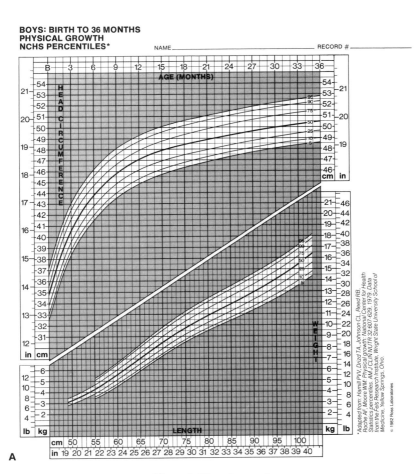

Figure 4–5A   *Continued*

Continued on following page.

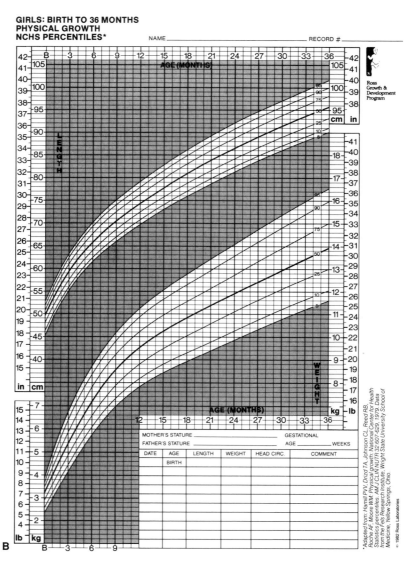

Figure 4–5B   The statistics for girls.

GIRLS: BIRTH TO 36 MONTHS
PHYSICAL GROWTH
NCHS PERCENTILES*

NAME _____ RECORD # _____

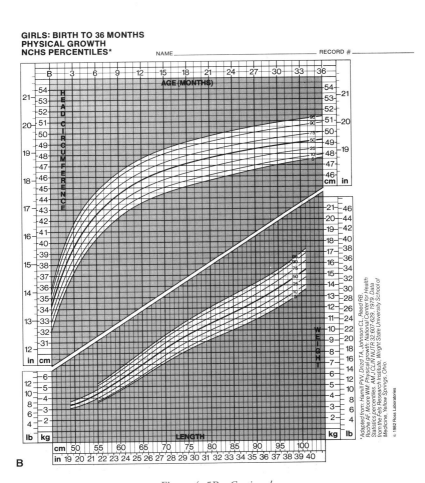

*Adapted from: Hamill PVV, Drizd TA, Johnson CL, Reed RB,
Roche AF, Moore WM: Physical growth: National Center for Health
Statistics percentiles. AM J CLIN NUTR 32:607-629 1979. Data
from the Fels Research Institute, Wright State University School of
Medicine, Yellow Springs, Ohio.
© 1982 Ross Laboratories

B

Figure 4–5B *Continued*

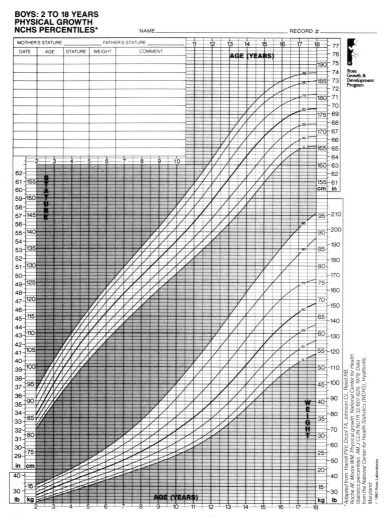

Figure 4–6A National Center for Health Statistics (NCHS) growth charts, ages 2 to 18 years. A, The NCHS percentiles for boys. (Figures provided through the courtesy of Ross Laboratories, Columbus, Ohio.)

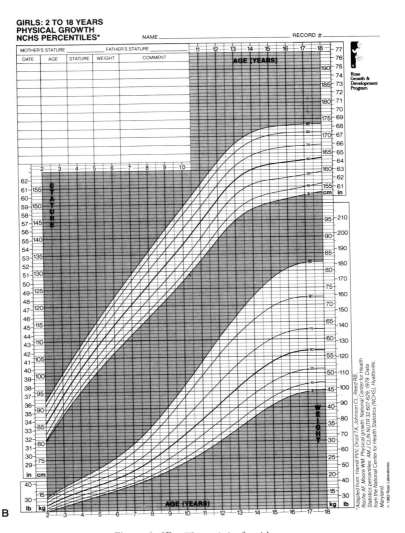

Figure 4–6B   The statistics for girls.

In a newborn infant, after the umbilical cord stump has fallen off, the examiner must check for an *umbilical granuloma,* which should be cauterized with silver nitrate.

Auscultate the abdomen (p. 370), percuss the abdomen (p. 371), and palpate the abdomen, using light and deep palpation (pp. 375–376). Are any masses present?

Palpate for the *liver, spleen,* and *kidneys* (pp. 376, 377, 379). The estimated liver span of a 6-month-old infant varies from 2.5 to 3.0 cm. At 1 year, the span is approximately 3 cm. The spleen is commonly palpable 1 to 2 cm below the left costal margin during the first month of life.

Genitalia

Inspect the external genitalia. Check for *ambiguous genitalia.* Is diaper rash present?

The foreskin is not fully retractable until 1 year of age. Diaper rash can cause *balanitis,* which is an acute inflammation of the glans penis. Boys who are uncircumcised may develop phimosis after balanitis.

Observe the position of the *urethral meatus.*

Inspect the *scrotum.* Is unilateral swelling present? Enlargement may represent a hernia or a hydrocele. Transilluminate any suspicious mass (pp. 409, 620). Auscultate a suspicious mass. Listening to a hernia containing bowel may reveal bowel sounds.

Palpate the testes. Are they both in the scrotum? Can an undescended testicle be palpated in the inguinal canal? If not, while the infant is lying on the examination table, you should press on the abdomen while trying to palpate the undescended testicle in the inguinal canal with the other hand.

In the female infant, is a *vaginal discharge* present? Commonly, there is a whitish, often blood-tinged discharge lasting for 1 month after birth. This is related to the placental transfer of maternal hormones.

Inspect the *perineum* for any rashes or lesions

Musculoskeletal Examination

Palpate the *clavicle.* At 1 month of age, the presence of a callus suggests a healed clavicular fracture.

The *hips* must be reexamined for dislocation at every routine visit for the first year of life (p. 620).

Neurologic Examination

By the fourth month, when the supine infant is pulled into a sitting position, no head lag should be present. By the eighth month, the infant should be able to sit without support.

Coordination of the hands begins at about 5 months of age, when infants can reach and grasps objects. By 7 months, they can transfer these objects from hand to hand. At 8 or 9 months, they should be able to use a pincer grip to pick up small objects.

Ears

The child can be either placed on the examination table or held by a parent. To examine the right ear, use your left hand to **pull the pinna out, back, and down** as the right hand holds the otoscope firmly against the child's forehead. Always use the largest speculum possible. The speculum is introduced slowly into the external canal (p. 620). The *tympanic membrane* should be easily visualized.

Is the tympanic membrane erythematous? Bulging? Check for a light reflex (p. 620). Are air-fluid levels visible behind the drum?

Mouth and Pharynx

The examination of the mouth and pharynx is the last part of the examination in this age group.

The child should be seated on the parent's lap, with the parent holding the child's head. The crying infant can usually be examined without the tongue depressor. The frightened child with the mouth firmly closed can be examined if you hold the child's nose; this will make the child open the mouth. The tongue depressor can then be slipped between the teeth over the tongue. Be quick if you must be foreceful.

Inspect the *gingivae.* Is gingival ulceration present (p. 621)?

Are any *teeth* present? The first teeth to erupt are the lower central incisors at about 6 months. These are followed by the lower lateral incisors at 7 months and the upper central teeth at 7 or 8 months. The upper lateral teeth begin to erupt at about 9 months. Increased salivation occurs temporarily with the eruption of new teeth (Table 4–3).

EXAMINATION OF THE YOUNG CHILD

The child who is 1 to 5 years of age needs to be relaxed for adequate examination. It is very important to children in this age group that you speak softly and that you demonstrate the parts of the examination on dolls or toy animals, on yourself, or on the parent. *Talk* to the child. It is amazing how easily an examination can often be per-

TABLE 4-3 Chronology of Dentition

| | Deciduous Teeth | | | | Permanent Teeth Eruption | |
	Eruption Maxillary (mo)	Eruption Mandibular (mo)	Shedding Maxillary (yr)	Shedding Mandibular (yr)	Maxillary (yr)	Mandibular (yr)
Central incisors	6–8	5–7	7–8	6–7	7–8	6–7
Lateral incisors	8–11	7–10	8–9	7–8	8–9	7–8
Canines	16–20	16–20	11–12	9–11	11–12	9–11
First premolars	—	—	—	—	10–11	10–12
Second premolars	—	—	—	—	10–12	11–13
First molars	10–16	10–16	10–11	10–12	6–7	6–7
Second molars	20–30	20–30	10–12	11–13	12–13	12–13
Third molars	—	—	—	—	17–22	17–22

formed by telling the young child a simple fantasy about imaginary animals. Ask the child questions about these characters. A reassuring voice goes a long way in making the child comfortable. Children less than 3 years of age are best examined on the parent's lap (p. 621).

The child should be completely undressed for the examination. If the child is modest, remove only the clothing that is necessary for the examination. Modesty varies greatly among children in this age group. Respect the child's modesty!

Start the examination by washing your hands in warm water. In addition to being clean, the warm hands are more comfortable for the child. If the child is on an examination table, have the parent stand at the child's feet. Any child in respiratory distress is easiest to examine in the position of most comfort, usually sitting or lying prone.

The child should always be told what to do instead of being asked to do something (p. 621).

In a child who appears to be *uncooperative,* auscultation of the heart and lungs should be performed *first,* because this requires the child's cooperation and should be performed early, when the child may be more cooperative. Because the sight of medical instruments is likely to frighten a child, use them last. Proceed with the examination in the following order for the *cooperative* child:

- **Take measurements**
- **Inspect the skin**
- **Examine the head**
- **Inspect the feet and hands**
- **Examine the neck**
- **Examine the chest**
- **Examine the heart**
- **Examine the abdomen**
- **Examine the genitalia**
- **Examine the eyes**
- **Examine the nose**
- **Examine the ears**
- **Examine the mouth and pharynx**
- **Measure blood pressure, if indicated**
- **Assess deep tendon reflexes, if indicated**
- **Take the temperature, if indicated**

General Assessment

The heart rate of a child 1 to 5 years of age ranges from 80 to 140 beats/min; the average rate is 100. The respiratory rate varies between 30 and 40 breaths/min.

Blood pressure assessment by auscultation is usually possible with children more than 3 or 4 years of age and should be performed on all children (p. 295). It is important to inform the child that the cuff will get tight for a few moments. The size of the cuff is important. The cuff must cover two thirds of the distance between the antecubital fossa and the shoulder. A cuff that is too small will result in falsely high readings; conversely, a cuff that is too large will result in readings that are falsely low (Fig. 4–7) (p. 622).

Determine the *height, weight,* and *head circumference,* and plot these values on the standard growth charts.

Skin

The examination of the skin is the same for children as for adults.

Carefully describe any rash present.

Examine the spine. Are tufts of hair along the spine, especially over the sacrum, present? These may mark the location of *spina bifida occulta.*

Is there evidence of *trauma* or *child abuse* (p. 617)?

Head

Examine the *lymph nodes* (p. 141).

Inspect the *shape of the head.*

Palpate the *sutures* in the 1- to 3-year-old child. Are they depressed? Elevated?

Palpate over the *frontal* and *maxillary sinuses* in children older than the age of 2 years for any tenderness.

Inspect the area of the *parotid glands* for swelling. Palpate the area.

Musculoskeletal Examination

Observe the *gait* by telling the child to walk back and forth with shoes or socks on (p. 623).

Tell the child to stand in front of you, and inspect the legs. Is bowing present (p. 623)?

The child with a *limp* should be examined for evidence of trauma or localized bone tenderness (pp. 623–624).

The Trendelenburg test should be performed if weakness of the gluteus medius is suspected (Fig. 4–8) (p. 475).

Inspect the child's shoes. Is there evidence of abnormal wear?

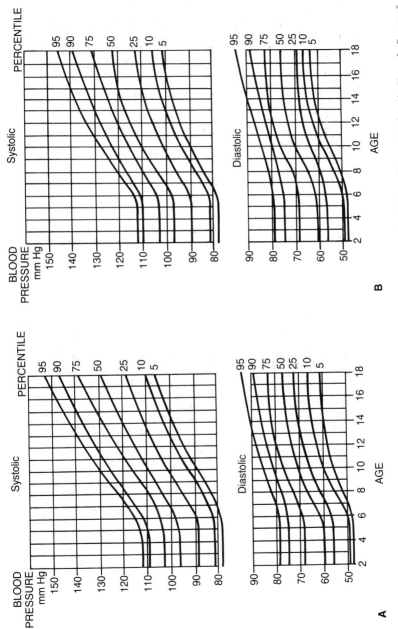

Figure 4–7 National Heart, Lung, and Blood Institute blood pressure measurements. *A*, Percentiles for boys. *B*, Percentiles for girls. (From the Report of the Task Force on Blood Pressure Control in Children of the National Heart, Lung, and Blood Institute. Reproduced by permission of Pediatrics (Suppl) 59:803, 1977.)

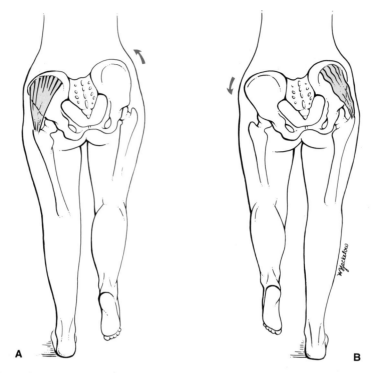

Figure 4–8   The Trendelenburg test. *A*, Position of the hips when subject is standing on the normal left leg. Notice that the right hip elevates as a result of contraction of the left hip musculature. *B*, Position of the hips when standing on the abnormal right leg. Notice that the left hip falls as a result of lack of adequate contraction of the right hip muscles.

Neurologic Examination

The development of speech, reading abilities, and the ability to manipulate small objects, throw a ball, and understand simple directions are the best indicators of a normally developing neurologic system.

Deep tendon reflexes are generally not tested unless there is reason to suspect that there may be a developmental abnormality (pp. 530, 531, 532).

Neck

Inspect the size and shape of the neck. Check for a *thyroglossal duct cyst* (p. 624).

Palpate the anterior and posterior triangles for lymphadenopathy (pp. 141, 624).

Palpate the *sternocleidomastoid muscle.*

Inspect the location of the *trachea.* Is it midline (p. 267)?

Palpate the *thyroid gland.* This is usually best felt with the child in a supine position. Use your thumb and index fingers to feel for the gland.

Chest

Inspect the shape of the chest (p. 259).

Determine the *respiratory rate.* The respiratory rate of a 6-year-old child is 16 to 20 breaths per minute.

Palpate the chest for tenderness (pp. 262–263). Tactile fremitus is a technique of low sensitivity in childhood.

Percuss the chest (p. 264). Because the chest wall is thinner in children than in adults, the percussion notes are more resonant in children than in adults. Percuss gently, because overly vigorous percussion may produce vibrations over a large area and obscure an area of dullness.

Auscultation is best performed by listening to the child when he or she is unaware of this portion of the examination. Telling a child to "take a deep breath" frequently results in the child's holding the breath. With a cooperative child, you can hold the youngster's nose while telling him or her to breathe in and out. Are the breath sounds normal? Are there any adventitious sounds? Breath sounds in the child sound louder than in the adult as a result of the chest's configuration.

Heart

In the cardiac examination of the young child, follow these procedures:

1. Inspect the precordium.
2. Palpate for any lifts, heaves, or thrills (pp. 303–306).
3. Auscultate in the four cardiac areas (pp. 306–310). Describe any murmurs or abnormal sounds.

Abdomen

Inspect the abdomen (p. 625).

Inspect the *umbilicus.* Tell the child to cough. Are there any bulging masses at the umbilicus?

Auscultate for peristaltic sounds. Are any *bruits* present (p. 625)? Percuss the abdomen for abnormal dullness.

Assess by light palpation (pp. 375–376). Is tenderness noted? Observe the patient's face during palpation.

Assess by deep palpation (p. 376).

Palpate the *liver* and *spleen* (pp. 376–379). The liver span of a 3-year-old is approximately 4 cm. By 5 years of age, the span has increased to 5 cm.

Palpate the *kidneys* by ballottement (p. 625). Place your left hand under the right costal margin at the costovertebral angle. Your right hand is placed over the midposition of the right abdomen. Tap firmly on the abdomen to try to feel the size of the kidney. The hands should be reversed to feel the left kidney.

Palpate the *femoral pulses*. Place the tips of your fingers along the inguinal ligament, midway between the symphysis pubis and the iliac crest. Time the pulse with the radial pulse; they should peak at the same time.

Palpate the femoral *lymph nodes*. It is common to find several 0.5 to1.0 cm nodes.

Inspect the *anus*. Is diaper rash present? Is there evidence of excoriations (p. 625)?

Rectal examination is usually not part of the standard examination in this age group. Only children with abdominal pain or symptoms referable to the lower gastrointestinal tract require a rectal examination. Instruct the child to lie on his or her back and flex the knees. Tell the child that the examination will be like "taking your temperature." You should use your fifth finger, gloved and well lubricated, for the examination. Tenderness and sphincter tone are determined, as well as the presence of any mass.

Genitalia

If the child is male, inspect the *penis*. Check for *phimosis*. By the end of the first year, the foreskin can be retracted in most uncircumcised boys. By the age of 4 years, the foreskin should be easily retractable in 80% of all uncircumcised boys.

Inspect the *urethral meatus*.

Inspect the *scrotum*. Is there any unilateral enlargement present? If the scrotum appears large, transilluminate and auscultate the scrotum (p. 626).

Palpate the *testicles* (p. 626). Are both present in the scrotum? In this age group, the testicles are often retracted into the inguinal canal. If one or both testicles are not felt in the scrotum, tell the child to sit on a chair with his feet on the seat. Instruct him to grab his knees. Repeat the palpation. This additional abdominal pressure may force a retracted or undescended testicle into the scrotum. Warm hands and a warm room often aid in this procedure.

Another useful maneuver to counteract an active cremasteric reflex is to have the child lie down and flex his leg at the knee, placing his foot on the opposite leg. This "tailor position" will bring the tendon of the sartorius muscle over the inguinal canal and prevent an active reflex from retracting the testicle.

Palpation for an *inguinal hernia* can usually be performed in children aged 4 years or older. The procedure is the same as in adults (pp. 410–411).

In the female patient, inspect the *vaginal area.* Is a *rash* present? Rashes in this area may be related to bubble baths. Is a *discharge* present? A discharge in girls aged 2 to 6 years is commonly related to a vaginal foreign body. A nasal speculum is often used to inspect the vagina for the cause of the discharge. Look for an intact hymen and a smooth vaginal opening. Be on the lookout for sexual abuse. The most important signs of abuse include difficulty in walking, vaginal or anal infections, genital irritation or swelling, torn or stained underclothes, vaginal or anal bleeding, and bruises.

Eyes

Visual acuity in children 1 to 3 years of age is assessed by their ability to identify brightly colored objects and by their ability to circumnavigate the examining room. Further visual acuity testing may be performed by using the Snellen eye chart and asking the child which way the letter faces: up, down, to the right, to the left. Visual acuity for a 3-year-old child is 20/40; at age 4 or 5 years, it is 20/30.

Confrontation visual field testing is performed only in children more than 4 years of age in whom there is a suspicion of decreased acuity. The test is conducted as in adults except that a small toy is used instead of finger counting (p. 160). The toy is brought in from the periphery of the child's vision, and the child is instructed to tell the examiner when he or she sees it.

Check *ocular motility.* Are the eyes straight? Be aware that the child with large epicanthal folds that partially cover the globe may be thought to have strabismus. The eyes should be parallel in all fields of gaze. Shine a light from 2 feet away and have the child look at it. The light should fall in the center of both pupils. Hold the patient's head and turn it to the right and then to the left while the position of the light is maintained. Is the corneal reflection symmetric in both eyes as the head is turned? If there is asymmetry, perform the *cover test* (p. 162).

Is the eye red (p. 626)?

Nose

Inspect the nostrils. Is flaring of the nostrils, associated with respiratory distress, present?

Inspect the tip of the nose. Is there a permanent transverse crease near the lower part of the nose when the tip is directed upward? This is commonly seen in allergy sufferers. This unmistakable sign of an allergy sufferer is caused by the *allergic salute:* using a palm or an extended forefinger to rub the nose upward and outward.

Elevate the tip of the nose and inspect the nasal mucosa. Are secretions present? If present, describe them (p. 626).

Check for *nasal polyps* (p. 626).

Ears

Is any *discharge* present? If so, describe it (p. 627).

Use the otoscope (p. 627) to inspect the *external canal* and *tympanic membrane.* A cooperative 2- to 3-year-old child may be either sitting or lying prone on the examination table, with the head turned to one side. An uncooperative child can be held in a parent's arms or lying prone. Insert the speculum tip to only ½ inch.

Inspect the tympanic membrane. Is it erythematous? Is it bulging? Is the tympanic membrane perforated? Does the tympanic membrane move with insufflation (p. 627)?

Palpate the *mastoid tip.* Tenderness is suggestive of mastoiditis.

Are *posterior auricular lymph nodes* present (pp. 141, 627)?

Check *hearing.* Hearing is necessary for normal development of language beyond the one-word stage. As a screening test, occlude one ear and whisper a number into the child's other ear. Ask the child to say the number that he or she heard. Repeat the test with the other ear. If a hearing loss is suspected, perform the Weber and Rinne tests (pp. 204–206). If there is a hearing loss, the child should be scheduled for audiometric testing as soon as possible.

Mouth and Pharynx

The evaluation of the mouth and pharynx is usually the last part of the examination of the small child.

Inspect the *lips* for any lesions and color.

Say to the child: "Open your mouth. I am going to count your teeth."

Count the number of *teeth* and inspect them for caries. The first lower molars erupt at the age of about 1 year. These are followed by the first upper molars at 14 months, lower cuspids at 16 months, upper cuspids at 18 months, second lower molars at 20 months, and finally the second upper molars at 2 years. This completes the primary dentition of 20 teeth. Flattened edges are seen in children who grind their teeth (p. 627).

Inspect the *bite*. Maxillary protrusion is termed *overbite* and is the normal position; mandibular protrusion is termed *underbite*. Have the child bite down while you inspect the occlusion. Normally, the upper teeth override the lower teeth.

Inspect the *gingivae* for any lesions.

Inspect the *buccal mucosa* (p. 628).

Inspect the *tongue*. Geographic tongue is a normal variation (p. 628).

The child should be seated during this part of the examination for best visualization of the posterior pharynx. Tell the youngster that you are going to look into his or her throat and that he or she should open the mouth as widely as possible. If the child is uncooperative, lay him or her down on the back on the examination table. The parent should stand at the head of the table. The child's hands are raised over the head, and the parent squeezes the child's elbows against the head so that the head does not move. The examiner can then lean over the child, holding a tongue blade in one hand and a light in the other.

Inspect the *posterior pharynx*. Inspect the size of the *tonsils*. Tonsillar size is estimated on a scale from 1+ to 4+, 4+ indicating that the tonsils meet in the midline. Is a purulent exudate present? Is a membrane present (p. 628)?

Are *petechiae* present (p. 628)?

Inspect the *posterior pharyngeal wall* (p. 628).

EXAMINATION OF THE OLDER CHILD

Children aged 6 to 12 years are usually a pleasure to examine. They understand the purpose of the examination and rarely present any problems. It is often very helpful to engage a child in conversation regarding school, friends, and hobbies. Conversation will help to relax the child even if the child does not appear apprehensive.

Allow the child to wear a gown or drape.

The order of the examination is essentially the same as in adults. If the child is complaining of pain in a certain area, that area should be examined last. As with younger children, brief explanations about each part of the examination should be given to older children.

It is important that you wash your hands with soap and warm water before beginning the examination.

General Assessment

In children 6 to 12 years of age, the *temperature* may be taken orally. The pulse of an average child in this age group varies from 75 to 125 beats/min, and the respirations vary from 15 to 20 breaths/min.

Blood pressure should be obtained in all children in this age group (pp. 295–296). It is very important to use the correct cuff size.

Measure the height and weight, and chart these on the child's record.

Skin

Inspect the skin for any evidence of fungal disease, especially between the toes.

Are any *rashes* present? Persistent dandruff may be tinea and not seborrhea. Seborrhea is commonly seen in infancy and adolescence.

Eyes

The examination of the eyes is essentially the same as in adults, with emphasis on *visual acuity.* A careful test with a standard Snellen eye chart is necessary (p. 159).

Ears

The examination of the ears is as in adults, with emphasis on *auditory acuity* (pp. 203–204). Audiometric testing should be performed on all school-aged children.

Nose

Examine the nose (pp. 209–212).

Mouth and Pharynx

The *teeth* should be carefully examined with respect to their condition and spacing. Have the child bite down, and observe the *bite* (p. 629).

Inspect the *tongue* for dryness, size, and any lesions. Deep furrows are common and have no clinical significance.

Inspect the *palate* for petechiae.

Inspect the *tonsils* for enlargement, injection, and exudation.

Neck

Palpate the *thyroid* for nodules (p. 142). The thyroid is rarely palpable in normal children in this age group.

Palpate for *lymphadenopathy* (p. 141).

Is the *trachea* at midline (pp. 267–269)?

Chest

The examination of the chest is the same as in adults (pp. 259–270).

Heart

The examination of the heart is the same as in adults (pp. 290–311).

Abdomen

The order of the abdominal examination is the same as in adults (pp. 363–380). The span of the liver at age 8 years is 5.0 to 5.5 cm; at age 12 years, the span is approximately 5.5 to 6.5 cm.

Genitalia

The age at development of the secondary sexual characteristics varies greatly. Development of the breast in girls may begin as early as age 8 years and continues for the next 5 years. The development of pubic hair in girls occurs at the same time. Testicular development in boys begins somewhat later, at about 9 or 10 years of age. Pubic hair starts to develop in boys at about age 12 years and continues to develop until age 15. The growth of the penis begins about a year after the beginning of testicular enlargement, at age 10 or 11 years. Whereas the growth spurt of girls occurs at about age 12, this spurt is not seen until around age 14 years in boys.

Sex maturity ratings for boys and girls have been established by Tanner. In the boy, the growth of pubic hair and the development of the penis, testes, and scrotum are used to assign sex maturity rating in values from 1 to 5. The examiner should record two ratings, one rating for the pubic hair and the other rating for the genitalia. If the development of the penis differs from that of the testes and scrotum, the two ratings should be averaged (Figs. 4–9 and 4–10, *A*).

The sex maturity ratings for girls are based on the growth of pubic hair and the development of the breasts. Five stages are also observed for each. The examiner should record two ratings, one for the breasts and the other for the pubic hair (Figs. 4–10, *B* and 4–11).

The youngster should be given a gown to avoid embarrassment in front of a parent.

Genital Development Stages: Boys

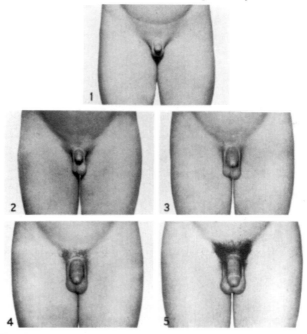

Stage	Characteristics
1	Prepubertal. Testes, scrotum, and penis are about the same size and proportion as in early childhood.
2	Enlargement of the testes and scrotum. Scrotal skin reddens and coarsens. Little change in size of penis.
3	Enlargement of penis, which occurs mainly in length. Further growth of testes and scrotum.
4	Further enlargement of penis with growth in width and length. Enlargement of glans penis. Scrotal skin darkens.
5	Adult genitalia.

Figure 4–9   Genital development in boys. Numbers indicate sex maturity ratings. (Reprinted with permission from Tanner JM: *Growth at Adolescence*, 2nd ed. Oxford, England, Blackwell Scientific Publications, Ltd., 1962.)

Inspect the *external genitalia*. Is *pubic hair* present? What are the *Tanner sex maturity ratings?* Are any lesions present? Is there evidence of sexual abuse (p. 617)?

Palpate the testes. Is an *inguinal hernia* present?

Pelvic examinations are not routine in this age group, unless clinically indicated (p. 633).

Pubic Hair Stages: Boys and Girls

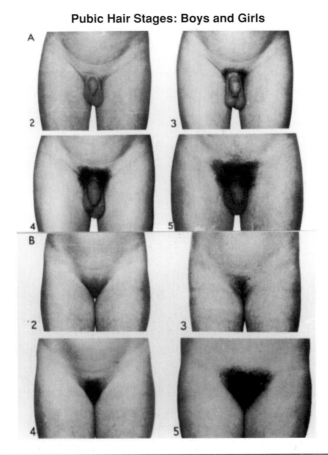

Stage	Characteristics
1	Prepubertal. No true pubic hair.
2	Sparse growth of slightly pigmented, downy hair. Only slightly curled. Hair mainly at base of penis or along labia.
3	Increase in hair, which is becoming coarser, curled, and darker.
4	Adult-type hair, but limited in area. No spread to medial surface of thighs.
5	Adult-type hair with spread to thighs.

Figure 4–10   Pubic hair development. *A*, Development in boys. *B*, Development in girls. Numbers indicate sex maturity ratings. (Reprinted with permission from Tanner JM: Growth at Adolescence, 2nd ed. Oxford, England, Blackwell Scientific Publications, Ltd., 1962.)

Breast Development Stages: Girls

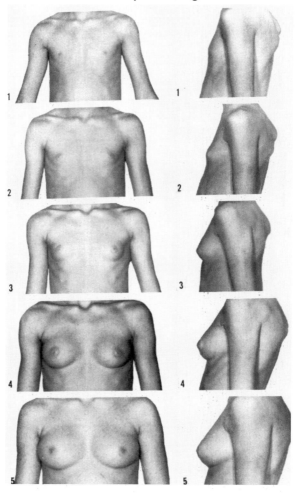

Stage	Characteristics
1	Prepubertal. Elevation of only papilla.
2	Breast bud stage. Elevation of breast and papilla as a small mound. Enlargement of diameter of areola.
3	Further enlargement of breast and areola with no separation of contours.
4*	Areola projected above level of breast as a secondary mound.
5	Mature stage. Recession of areola mound to the general contour of the breast. Projection of papilla only.

*This stage does not occur in all girls. In approximately 25% of girls, it is absent. In addition, many adult women have a persistence of this stage throughout life.

Musculoskeletal Examination

The most important part of the musculoskeletal examination of children aged 6 to 12 is for detection of *scoliosis*. Scoliosis is the most common spinal deformity, especially in pubertal girls. Have the patient stand stripped to the waist. Inspect the back. Are the shoulders or scapulae at the same height? Is the occiput aligned over the intergluteal cleft? Ask the child to bend down and try to touch the toes, allowing the arms to hang freely. A unilateral elevation of the lower ribs is seen in patients with scoliosis (Fig. 4–12). Another, similar method of detecting scoliosis is to mark the spinous processes with a pen while the child is standing in front of you. Then ask the child to bend forward from the waist. A deviation of the marks to either side suggests scoliosis. Unfortunately, none of the methods of detecting scoliosis has been shown to have adequate sensitivity or specificity (pp. 633–634).

Neurologic Examination

In children of this age group, the complete neurologic examination is indicated only when there is evidence of developmental abnormalities. Ths neurologic examination is essentially the same as in the adult patient.

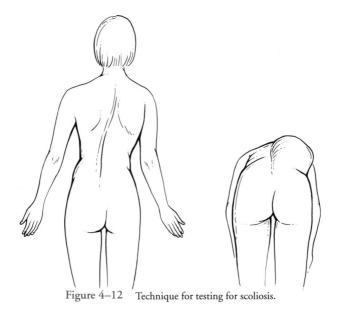

Figure 4–12   Technique for testing for scoliosis.

Figure 4–11   Breast development in girls. Numbers indicate sex maturity ratings. (Reprinted with permission from Tanner JM: Growth at Adolescence, 2nd ed. Oxford, England, Blackwell Scientific Publications, Ltd., 1962.)

EXAMINATION OF THE ADOLESCENT

The examination of adolescents is exactly the same as that of the adult patient. It is appropriate for the examiner to ask the parent to leave during the examination and perhaps even for the history.

Because the examination is so similar to that of adults, only the dissimilarities are described in this section.

General Assessment

Assess *heart rate*. The average heart rate of the adolescent is 60 to 100 beats/min.

Assess *respiratory rate*. The respiratory rate varies from 12 to 18 respirations/min by age 16 years.

Assess *blood pressure* (pp. 295–298).

Skin

Examination of the skin of adolescents usually reveals evidence of *pubertal changes*. These include acne, areolar pigmentation, functioning of the apocrine sweat glands, pigmentation of the external genitalia, and the development of axillary and pubic hair.

Breast

Determine the *Tanner sex maturity rating* of the breasts in girls (pp. 629–633).

Breast development occurs in both boys and girls. The boy with unilateral gynecomastia should be reassured that this change is part of normal puberty and will be transient.

Asymmetric breast development in girls is common. Reassure the patient that puberty is progressing normally.

Abdomen

The abdominal examination is the same as in the adult. The liver span of a 16-year-old adolescent varies from 6 to 7 cm.

Genitalia

Determine the *sex maturity ratings* of the pubic hair and genitalia for male patients (pp. 629–633). Determine the sex maturity rating of the pubic hair for female patients.

The examiner should evaluate the patient carefully and try to reassure him or her that the body changes are related to normal puberty.

If an internal pelvic examination of the female adolescent is necessary, an extremely gentle approach is required. The use of a Pedersen speculum often makes the examination less uncomfortable. A female nurse is always required to be present if the examiner is male (pp. 433–437).

Musculoskeletal Examination

Knee pain in the adolescent is usually the result of trauma. Partial avulsion of the tibial tubercle associated with a painful swelling in that area is called *Osgood-Schlatter disease.* This common condition is seen more commonly in pubertal boys and is usually self-limited.

The Clinical Evaluation of a Pregnant Patient

CHAPTER 5

Taking a Comprehensive History from a Pregnant Patient

It was the best of times, it was the worst of times . . .
Charles Dickens
1812–1870

Any woman of reproductive age who has symptoms, even if not directly related to the abdomen, should be evaluated for pregnancy. *"Think pregnancy"* should be your motto in the evaluation of this patient (p. 563). This is extremely important because the diagnosis or treatment of her medical or surgical problem may be deleterious to her developing fetus, if indeed she is pregnant. Many of the symptoms of pregnancy are nonspecific and could be interpreted erroneously if the pregnancy is not recognized.

COMMON SYMPTOMS OF PREGNANCY

The most common symptoms of pregnancy are amenorrhea, nausea, breast changes, heartburn, backache, abdominal enlargement, quickening, skin and nail changes, disturbances in urination, vaginal discharge, and fatigue.

Amenorrhea (p. 569)
Nausea (p. 569)

Nausea, with or without vomiting, is the so-called *morning sickness of pregnancy.* The pregnant woman is also hypersensitive to odors, and she may experience alterations in taste. Morning sickness usually abates after 12 to 16 weeks. Severe vomiting may result in dehydration and ketosis.

Breast Changes (p. 569)

One of the earliest symptoms of pregnancy is an **increase in the vascularity of the breast** associated with a sensation of **heaviness,** almost pain. This occurs at about the sixth week. By the eighth week, the **nipple and areola have become more pigmented,** and the nipple becomes more erectile. The **Montgomery tubercles become prominent** as raised, pinkish red nodules on the areola. By the sixteenth week, a clear fluid called **colostrum** is secreted and may be expressed from the nipple. By the twentieth week, further pigmentation and mottling of the areola have developed (Fig. 5–1).

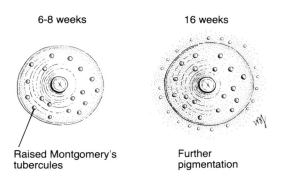

6-8 weeks   16 weeks

Raised Montgomery's tubercules   Further pigmentation

Figure 5–1   Breast changes during pregnancy.

Heartburn (p. 569)
Backache (p. 569)
Abdominal Enlargement (p. 570)

The uterus rises out of the pelvis and into the abdomen by the twelfth week of gestation, and an increase in abdominal girth is usually apparent by the fifteenth week. This enlargement is usually more apparent earlier in multiparous women, in whom some of the tone of the abdominal muscles was lost in previous pregnancies.

Quickening (p. 570)

Quickening is the sensation of fetal movement. It is a very faint sensation initially. Quickening usually begins at 20 weeks in the primigravida but is felt 2 to 3 weeks earlier in the multipara.

Skin and Nail Changes (p. 570)

Hyperpigmentation is very common, especially in women with dark hair and a dark complexion. Areas prone to friction (e.g., medial aspect of thighs, axillae) also tend to darken. New pigmentation on the face, called **chloasma,** also commonly develops on the cheeks, forehead, nose, and chin. "Stretch marks," or **striae gravidarum,** are irregular, linear, pinkish purple lesions that develop on the abdomen, breasts, upper arms, buttocks, and thighs (Fig. 5–2).

In addition to skin changes, there may be **transverse grooving of the nails,** as well as increased brittleness or softening. **Eccrine sweating** progressively increases throughout pregnancy, whereas apocrine gland activity decreases. **Hirsutism** may also occur on the face, arms, legs, and back.

Disturbances in Urination (p. 570)

Beginning at the sixth week, urinary bladder symptoms, such as increased **frequency of urination,** are common. As the uterus rises above the pelvis, the symptoms tend to

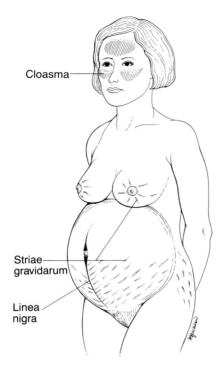

Cloasma

Striae gravidarum

Linea nigra

Figure 5–2   Common skin changes during pregnancy.

remit. Near term, however, urinary symptoms recur as the fetal head settles into the maternal pelvis and impinges on the volume capacity of the urinary bladder.

Vaginal Discharge (p. 571)

An asymptomatic, white, milky vaginal discharge is common.

Fatigue (p. 572)
Other Symptoms

Other symptoms include *varicose veins, headache, leg cramps, swelling of the legs and hands, constipation, bleeding gums, insomnia, and "dizziness."*

OBSTETRIC RISK ASSESSMENT

The medical history of the pregnant woman is similar to that of the nonpregnant woman. In addition, the interviewer must carefully assess obstetric risk. The following major risk factors must be evaluated: age, parity, height, pregnancy weight, diabetes, hypertension, renal disease, hemoglobinopathy and isoimmunization, history of previous pregnancies, sexually transmitted infections, other infections, and tobacco, alcohol, and drug use.

Age

Older women have an increased risk of conceiving fetuses with chromosomal abnormalities (p. 572).

Parity

Women who have had more than five children are at greater risk of *placenta previa* and *placenta accreta.* Postpartum hemorrhage and uterine rupture are also more common in this group of women (p. 572).

Height

Women who are less than 5 feet tall generally have a small pelvis and therefore may be prone to *cephalopelvic disproportion* (CPD), which may result in the need for a cesarean delivery.

Pregnancy Weight

The perinatal mortality rate is higher among women whose initial prepregnancy weight is less than 120 pounds, especially if their weight gain during pregnancy is less than 11 pounds.

History of Diabetes, Hypertension, or Renal Disease

Women with diabetes, hypertension, or renal disease are at an increased risk of fetal intrauterine growth retardation (IUGR), premature labor, toxemia, and abruptio placentae (p. 573).

Hemoglobinopathy and Isoimmunization

It is important to determine the presence of any hemoglobinopathy because pregnancy can precipitate an exacerbation of the anemia. Women who are Rh-negative must be monitored closely throughout pregnancy if they have Rh antibodies as a result of *isoimmunization,* because severe hemolytic anemia may develop in the fetus before delivery (p. 573).

History of Previous Pregnancies

A history of traumatic or second trimester abortions increases the possibility of cervical injury and subsequent incompetence of the cervix—an often preventable cause of second trimester miscarriage. A history of premature delivery (newborn's weight less than 2500 g) or immature delivery (less than 1000 g) increases the probability of recurrent early delivery. These patients require particularly close surveillance. A history of unexplained pregnancy loss in the third trimester should alert one to undiagnosed medical problems in the mother, such as gestational diabetes or systemic lupus erythematosus. Previous cesarean section requires exact information as to the reason for the procedure and the type of uterine incision used if the examiner is to make a proper assessment of whether a patient is a candidate for a vaginal birth after a previous cesarean (VBAC).

Sexually Transmitted Infections

Because medical treatment of the HIV-positive mother can reduce the rate of transmission of the infection to the fetus by more than two thirds, it is obvious that identification of the HIV-positive mother is essential. Although HIV testing cannot be required of the mother, it is mandatory that she be counseled about the value of testing. A history of genital herpes simplex will require screening for recurrences near the time of delivery, as these may necessitate cesarean delivery to prevent transmission to the neonate.

Other Infections

Careful questioning regarding exposure to rubella, chickenpox, or parvovirus (fifth disease) is critical. Antibody titers may be necessary to determine immunity.

Tobacco, Alcohol, and Drug Use

Inquire about the use of tobacco, alcohol, and recreational drugs, exposure to toxic substances in the workplace or at home, and exposure to other teratogenic agents. Women who smoke cigarettes place their fetus at a higher risk of complications and should be encouraged to stop. The fetus is more likely to exhibit IUGR and to have hypoxia during labor. Special note must be made of *any* drugs taken during pregnancy. Ideally, this information should be obtained before the woman conceives so that she can be counseled properly (p. 573).

• • •

A question that most women ask after being told that they are pregnant is, When am I due? To calculate the *expected date of confinement* (EDC), first determine the date of the onset of the last menstrual period (LMP) and then calculate the EDC as in the example below:

- LMP: 12/29/97
- Go back 3 months: 9/29/97
- Add 1 year: 9/29/98
- Add 7 days: 10/06/98 = EDC

Alternatively, the EDC can be calculated by adding 9 months and 7 days to the first day of the LMP. This calculation is based on a gestation of 280 days and is known as *Nägele's rule.* By knowing the EDC, the examiner can predict the size of the uterus on physical examination, provided that the LMP is correct and conception has actually occurred. If the size of the uterus differs significantly from that expected according to the EDC, the causes must be determined (pp. 573–574).

CHAPTER 6

The Physical Examination of a Pregnant Patient

The physician must generalize the disease, and individualize the patient.
Christopy Wilheim Hufeland
1762–1836

The equipment necessary for the examination of the pregnant woman is the same as for the nonpregnant woman. In addition, specialized instruments such as an ultrasonic scan, ultrasonic Doppler scan, or fetoscope may be used for listening to the fetal heart. The ultrasonic scan can detect the fetal heart beat as early as weeks 6 to 7; an ultrasonic Doppler scan is used at about week 10; and a fetoscope or stethoscope can be used after week 20 to auscultate the fetal heartbeat.

Always try to make the patient as comfortable as possible. She should be examined in comfortable surroundings with attention to privacy. Discuss with her all of the procedures that you will perform. The patient's gown should open in the front for ease of the examination. If the patient is in advanced pregnancy, avoid having her lie for a long period on her back. It is useful for the woman to urinate before the pelvic examination. As always, wash your hands before beginning the examination. Make sure that your hands are warm and dry!

Because the examination of the pregnant woman is identical to other examinations described in the chapter on the examination of an adult patient, only the special techniques and the modifications of the examination are discussed here.

THE INITIAL COMPREHENSIVE EVALUATION

Achieve three main goals in the initial evaluation:

1. **Determine the health of the mother and fetus.**
2. **Determine the gestational age of the fetus.**
3. **Initiate a plan for continuing care.**

The physical examination must include the following:

- **Determination of height and weight**
- **Assessment of blood pressure**
- **Inspection of the teeth and gums**
- **Palpation of the thyroid gland**
- **Auscultation of the heart and lungs**
- **Examination of the breasts and nipples**
- **Examination of the abdomen**
- **Examination of the legs for varicosities and edema**

121

- **Examination of the pelvis**
- **Inspection of the vagina and cervix**
- **Cytologic study (Pap smear)**
- **Swab for *Chlamydia* and gonorrhea**

Whenever possible, ultrasonography should be performed at about 16 to 20 weeks of gestation to confirm that the pregnancy is progressing normally, to check for multiple fetuses, to estimate precisely the maturity of the fetus, and to recognize any major abnormality.

Head, Eyes, Ears, Nose, Throat, and Neck

Inspect the *face*. Is chloasma present (p. 570)? What is the *texture of the hair and skin?*

Inspect the mouth (pp. 231–232). What is the *condition of the teeth and gums?*

Palpate the *thyroid* (p. 142). Is it enlarged symmetrically?

Chest

Inspect, palpate, percuss, and auscultate the *chest* (pp. 259–270). Is there any evidence of labored breathing?

Heart

Palpate for the *point of maximum impulse* (PMI) (p. 251). Is it displaced laterally?

Auscultate the heart (pp. 306–310). Systolic ejection murmurs are very common during pregnancy as a result of the hyperdynamic state. Diastolic murmurs are always pathologic!

Breasts

Inspect the breasts (p. 344). Are they symmetric? Notice the presence of vascular engorgement and pigmentary changes. Are the nipples everted? An inverted nipple may interfere with a woman's plans to breast-feed.

Palpate the breasts (pp. 347–349). The normal nodularity of breast tissue is accentuated during pregnancy, but *any discrete mass should be considered pathologic until proved otherwise.*

Abdomen

Inspect for the *linea nigra* and the *striae gravidarum* (p. 570). Notice the contour of the abdomen.

Palpate the abdomen (pp. 375–376). Fetal movement may be felt by the examiner after 24 weeks. Are uterine contractions present? Hold your hand on the abdomen as the uterus relaxes.

Assess the *fundal height* with a tape measure. The measurement should be taken in a straight line from the top of the symphysis pubis to the top of the fundus while the bladder is empty (Fig. 6–1). Between 18 and 32 weeks of gestation, the superior-inferior measurement, in centimeters, should equal the number of weeks of gestation. The uterus rises up and enters the abdomen at 12 weeks. It reaches the umbilicus at 24 weeks and is just under the costal margin by 36 weeks (p. 576).

Auscultate the fetal heart and determine the *fetal heart rate* (FHR). Note its location. Throughout pregnancy, the FHR is approximately 120 to 160 beats/min. Between weeks 12 and 18, the FHR is usually detected in the midline of the lower abdomen. After 30 weeks, the FHR is best heard over the fetal chest or back. Knowing the location of the fetal back is helpful in determining where to listen for the FHR.

Genitalia

Inspect the external genitalia (pp. 431–433). Are any lesions present?

Inspect the anus. Are varicosities present?

With gloves on, perform a speculum examination (pp. 433–437). Make sure that the speculum has been warmed in water. Inspect the cervix (pp. 435–436). A dusky blue color is characteristic of pregnancy and occurs by weeks 6 to 8 of gestation. Is the cervix dilated? Is so, fetal membranes may be seen within. Note the character of the vaginal secretions. Obtain (1) cytologic studies for a Pap test and (2) a swab for *Chlamydia* and gonorrhea organisms. As the speculum is removed, inspect the vaginal walls. The vagi-

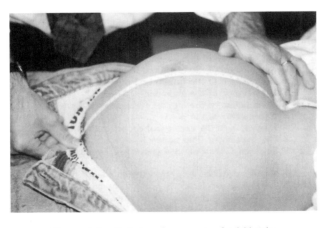

Figure 6–1　Technique for measuring fundal height.

nal walls are commonly blue-violaceous in pregnancy. Withdraw the speculum *carefully.*

Perform a *digital bimanual examination* (pp. 437–438), paying special attention to the following: the consistency, length, and dilation of the cervix; the fetal presenting part (in advanced pregnancy); the structure of the pelvis; and any abnormalities of the vagina and perineum. Is the cervix closed (p. 576)? Estimate the length of the cervix by palpating the lateral side of the cervix from the cervical tip to the lateral fornix. Only at term should the cervix shorten, or efface. The normal length of the cervix is 1.5 to 2.0 cm.

Palpate the uterus for size, consistency, and position (p. 438). Is *Hegar's sign* present (Fig. 6–2) (pp. 576–577)? Bimanual palpation of the uterus is useful up to about 12–14 weeks' gestation. After that, the uterus can be palpated abdominally. Fetal parts are usually palpated from about 26 to 28 weeks' gestation by abdominal examination.

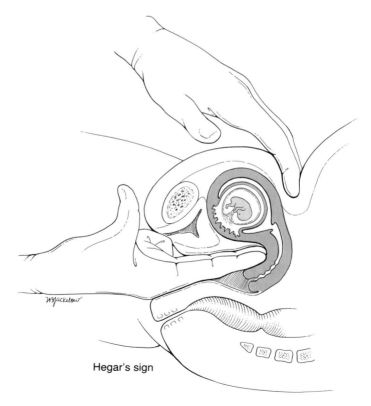

Hegar's sign

Figure 6–2   Technique for evaluating for the presence of Hegar's sign.

Palpate the adnexa (pp. 438–441). Early in pregnancy, the corpus luteum may be palpable as a cystic mass on one ovary. As you withdraw your hand from the vagina, evaluate the pelvic muscles.

A rectovaginal examination is **not** indicated unless the woman has a retroverted, retroflexed uterus.

Extremities

Inspect for varicosities (p. 331). Is edema present (pp. 310–311)?

This completes the routine initial examination.

SUBSEQUENT ANTENATAL EXAMINATIONS

Subsequent antenatal examinations are important for screening for impaired fetal growth, malpresentation, anemia, preeclampsia, and other problems. All parts of the examination indicated above are routinely performed during each visit. This section concerns, in particular, the abdominal examination.

The physical examination should confirm that fetal growth is consistent with gestational age. Attention should then be given to assessing the lie and the presentation of the fetus (pp. 565–568). From week 28 of gestation and on to term, the following four maneuvers, known as *Leopold's maneuvers,* provide vital information for the examiner. These maneuvers are performed with the woman lying on her back.

Perform the *first maneuver* to evaluate the upper pole and define the fetal part in the fundus of the uterus. Stand facing the patient at her side, and gently palpate the upper

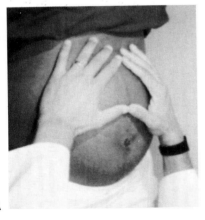

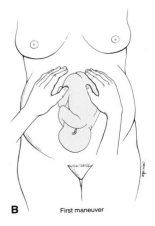

A   **B**   First maneuver

Figure 6–3   Leopold's first maneuver. *A,* Position of hands on abdomen. *B,* Illustration of relation of examiner's hands to fetus.

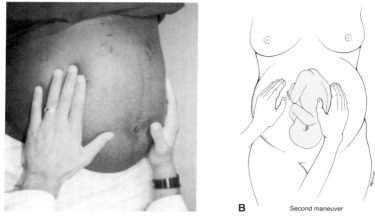

Figure 6–4   Leopold's second maneuver. *A,* Position of hands on abdomen. *B,* Illustration of relation of examiner's hands to fetus.

uterine fundus with your fingers to ascertain which fetal pole is present (Fig. 6–3). Usually, the fetal buttocks are felt at the upper pole. They feel firm but irregular. In a breech presentation, the head is at the upper pole. The head feels hard and round and is usually movable.

Perform the *second maneuver* to locate the position of the fetal back. Standing in the same place as with the first maneuver, place the palms of your hands on either side of the abdomen and apply gentle pressure to the uterus to identify the fetal back and

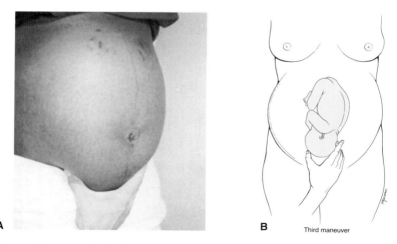

Figure 6–5   Leopold's third maneuver. Relation of hand and fetal presenting part. *A,* Position of hands on abdomen. *B,* Illustration of relation of examiner's hands to fetus.

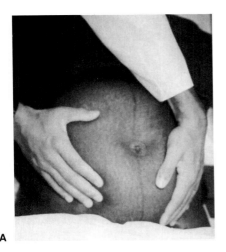
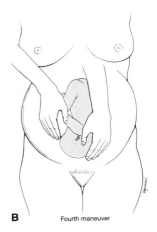

A   **B**   Fourth maneuver

Figure 6–6   Leopold's fourth maneuver. Relationship of hand and fetal presenting part. *A,* Position of hands on abdomen. *B,* Illustration of relation of examiner's hands to fetus. Note that the examiner's right hand is stopped higher by the cephalic prominence.

limbs (Fig. 6–4). On one side, the fetal back is felt: rounded, smooth, and hard. On the other side are the limbs, which are nodular or bumpy, and kicking may be felt.

Perform the *third maneuver* to palpate the lower pole of the fetus. From the same position as the first two maneuvers, use your thumb and fingers of one hand to grasp the lower portion of the maternal abdomen just above the symphysis pubis (Fig. 6–5). If the presenting portion is not engaged, a movable part, usually the head of the fetus, is felt. If the presenting portion is engaged, this maneuver indicates that the lower pole of the fetus is fixed in the pelvis.

Perform the *fourth maneuver* to confirm the presenting portion and to locate the side of the cephalic prominence. You should now stand beside the patient, facing her feet. Place your hands on either side of the lower abdomen. With the tips of your fingers, exert a deep pressure in the direction of the pelvic inlet (Fig. 6–6). If the presenting portion is the head and the head is flexed normally, one hand will be stopped sooner by the cephalic prominence, and the other hand will descend further into the pelvis. In a vertex presentation, the cephalic prominence is on the same side as the fetal small parts. In a vertex presentation with the head extended, the prominence is on the side of the back.

The Clinical Evaluation of a Geriatric Patient

CHAPTER 7

Taking a Comprehensive History from a Geriatric Patient

Old age isn't so bad when you consider the alternative.
Maurice Chevalier
1888–1972

The "geriatric patient" is a member of a group of individuals 65 years of age or older. The individuals in this group experience considerable variation in general health, mental status, functional ability, personal and social resources, marital status, living arrangements, creativity, and social integration. The age range of this rapidly growing population spans more than 40 years (p. 640).

One of the most important principles in geriatric medicine is the fact that patients may have an ***altered presentation of disease.*** The actual symptom may not be a symptom of the organ system involved with the disease (p. 645).

Another very important principle of geriatric medicine is the ***nonspecific presentation of disease.*** It is not uncommon that when an elderly person becomes ill, a family member reports that the patient "just hasn't gotten out of bed." The patient may go to bed and stay there. The patient may not want to eat and may have only nonspecific complaints.

A third principle is the ***underreporting of illness.*** When an interviewer asks a geriatric patient about various symptoms, the patient may fail to report blindness caused by a cataract, deafness caused by otosclerosis, pain in the legs at night, urinary incontinence, constipation, confusion, and so forth. The geriatric patient may actually believe that these symptoms are normal for a 75- or 80-year-old person (p. 646).

A fourth principle is the recognition that ***multiple pathologic conditions*** may be present in a geriatric patient. Such a patient may therefore have been given multiple medications or therapies. One medicine may have deleterious effects on a patient if some other condition also exists. Of course, this can occur with patients of any age, but it is more likely to occur in older patients, who probably have several pathologic conditions.

The fifth principle is that of ***polypharmacy,*** which is defined as the use of three or more medicines. It is critically important that the interviewer see and list all the medications being taken by the patient. Instruct the patient or family to bring in all medications, both prescription and nonprescription, and ask the patient how he or she is taking them (p. 646).

Finally, what is the patient's ***chief complaint?*** This is sometimes referred to as "the myth of the chief complaint." Many geriatric patients do not have just a single complaint. There may be several problems related to their many conditions. In fact, if a chief complaint is indeed given, it may bear no relation to the organ system involved.

Be careful in the evaluation of the chief complaint when dealing with the older patient (p. 646).

Expectations of geriatric patients are different from those of patients in other age groups. Whereas in younger patients the emphasis is on diagnosis and cure, the goal in the care of older patients is to improve function. You should strive to prolong the period of optimal physical, mental, and social activity. In the event of terminal illness, you should ensure as little mental and physical distress as possible and provide appropriate emotional support to the patient and family.

THE GERIATRIC HISTORY

The main components of the medical history are basically the same for geriatric patients as for younger patients, except for the chief complaint, which has already been discussed, and the family history. Except for a family history of Alzheimer's disease, the **family history is less important** in geriatric patients than in younger patients. For example, the fact that a family member died of a myocardial infarction at age 60 years is relatively unimportant for a patient who is already in his or her 80s! It is also often difficult for an older patient to remember the causes of and ages at death of relatives.

Before beginning the history, it is especially important to determine whether there is an **impairment of hearing, vision, or cognition.** A quick check of these three functions is mandatory. Ask the patient whether he or she uses any assistive devices (e.g., hearing aid, glasses, cane, walker, wheelchair). If so, evaluate the condition of the device. Is the patient using the device properly? Ask the patient how the device was obtained; often these devices have been given to the patient by friends or family members or have even been left by decreased spouses!

If a hearing impairment is determined, sit facing the patient, as close as possible and at ear level with the patient. Make sure that the patient is wearing, if required, the hearing aid or other assistive device. Try to minimize both audible and visual distractions. Speak in a slow, low-pitched, and moderately loud voice. Allow the patient to observe your lips as you talk. Finally, confirm with the patient that he or she is being understood by repeating portions of the history.

Because many older patients have a memory deficit or dementia, it is frequently necessary to obtain a **confirming history** from another family member or caregiver.

All support systems must be carefully evaluated. These include family, friends, and professional services.

It is extremely important to ascertain **diet**, because many older patients have a poorly balanced diet.

A *comprehensive geriatric assessment* is an essential component of the history. It ensures that the many complex health care needs are evaluated and met. Every geriatric history must include a comprehensive assessment of activities. Measures of the patient's ability to perform basic activities, called *activities of daily living (ADL),* must be gathered. These include measures of bathing, dressing, toileting, continence, feeding, and transferring in and out of bed or on and off a chair. The ability to perform more complex tasks, called *instrumental activities of daily living (IADL),* is also assessed. These tasks include food preparation, shopping, housekeeping, laundry, financial management, medicine management, use of transportation, and use of the telephone.

TABLE 7–1   Yesavage Geriatric Depression Scale

1. Are you basically satisfied with your life?	yes/no
2. Have you dropped many of your activities and interests?	yes/no
3. Do you feel that your life is empty?	yes/no
4. Do you often get bored?	yes/no
5. Are you hopeful about the future?	yes/no
6. Are you bothered by thoughts you can't get out of your head?	yes/no
7. Are you in good spirits most of the time?	yes/no
8. Are you afraid that something bad is going to happen to you?	yes/no
9. Do you feel happy most of the time?	yes/no
10. Do you often feel helpless?	yes/no
11. Do you often get restless and fidgety?	yes/no
12. Do you prefer to stay at home, rather than going out and doing new things?	yes/no
13. Do you frequently worry about the future?	yes/no
14. Do you feel you have more problems with memory than most?	yes/no
15. Do you think it is wonderful to be alive now?	yes/no
16. Do you often feel downhearted and blue?	yes/no
17. Do you feel pretty worthless the way you are now?	yes/no
18. Do you worry a lot about the past?	yes/no
19. Do you find life gets very exciting?	yes/no
20. Is it hard for you to get started on new projects?	yes/no
21. Do you feel full of energy?	yes/no
22. Do you feel that your situation is hopeless?	yes/no
23. Do you think that most people are better off than you are?	yes/no
24. Do you frequently get upset over little things?	yes/no
25. Do you frequently feel like crying?	yes/no
26. Do you have trouble concentrating?	yes/no
27. Do you enjoy getting up in the morning?	yes/no
28. Do you prefer to avoid social gatherings?	yes/no
29. Is it easy for you to make decisions?	yes/no
30. Is your mind as clear as it used to be?	yes/no

*Scoresheet**

1. No	2. Yes	3. Yes	4. Yes	5. No
6. Yes	7. No	8. Yes	9. No	10. Yes
11. Yes	12. Yes	13. Yes	14. Yes	15. No
16. Yes	17. Yes	18. Yes	19. No	20. Yes
21. No	22. Yes	23. Yes	24. Yes	25. Yes
26. Yes	27. No	28. Yes	29. No	30. No

Reprinted from Yesavage JA, Brink TL, Rose TL, et al.: Development and validation of a geriatic depression rating scale: A preliminary report. J Psychiatr Res *17*:37–49, 1983. Copyright 1983, with permission from Pergamon Press Ltd., Headington Hill Hall, Oxford OX3 0BW, United Kingdom.
*See *Textbook of Physical Diagnosis*, p. 648, for interpretation.

Inquire about a history of all of the following very important areas:

- **Abuse and neglect**
- **Affective disorder**
- **Caregiver stress**
- **Cognitive impairment**
- **Decubitus ulcers**
- **Dental impairment**
- **Discussion of advance directives** (i.e., living wills, resuscitation, and health proxy)
- **Falls**
- **Feeding impairment**
- **Gait abnormalities**
- **Health maintenance**
- **Hearing impairment**
- **Incontinence** (fecal and urinary)
- **Infections** (recurrent)
- **Nutritional assessment**
- **Osteoporosis**
- **Podiatric disorders**
- **Polypharmacy**
- **Preoperative evaluation**, if appropriate
- **Rehabilitation needs**
- **Sleep disorders**
- **Visual impairment**

Certain questionnaires and scales have been validated in elderly persons and may be used to *screen patients for affective disorders* such as depression or dementia. An example is the **Yesavage Geriatrics Depression Scale,** which consists of 30 items (Table 7–1) and in which each of the patient's answers that matches the scoresheet is scored 1 point. A total score between 0 and 9 indicates no depression; between 10 and 19, mild depression; and between 20 and 30, severe depression.

Finally, a careful *assessment of mental status* is required for all older patients. Memory deficits and decreased intellectual functioning influence the reliability of the medical history; therefore you must evaluate mental status early in your assessment. Casual conversation is rarely sufficient for detecting cognitive impairment in elderly persons. All older patients should be screened with the use of a validated instrument such as the **Folstein Mini-Mental State** (Table 7–2). A maximal score of 30 points is possible on this instrument. A score greater than 24 probably indicates no cognitive impairment. Patients with scores between 20 and 24 need further cognitive testing, unless educational, language, or cultural reasons are thought to play a role in the lowness of the score. Scores of less than 20 indicate cognitive impairment.

TABLE 7–2   Folstein's "Mini-Mental State"

Maximum Score	Score	
		Orientation
5	( )	What is the (year) (season) (date) (day) (month)?
5	( )	Where are we (state) (county) (town) (hospital) (floor)?
		Registration
3	( )	Name 3 objects: 1 second to say each. Then ask the patient all 3 after you have said them. Give 1 point for each correct answer. Then repeat them until he learns all 3. Count trials and record.
		Trials
		Attention and Calculation
5	( )	Serial 7's. 1 point for each correct. Stop after 5 answers. Alternatively, spell "world" backwards.
		Recall
3	( )	Ask for the 3 objects repeated above. Give 1 point for each correct.
		Language
9	( )	Name a pencil, and watch (2 points)
		Repeat the following "No ifs, ands or buts." (1 point)
		Follow a 3-stage command:
		"Take a paper in your right hand, fold it in half, and put it on the floor" (3 points)
		Read and obey the following:
		CLOSE YOUR EYES (1 point)
		Write a sentence (1 point)
		Copy design (1 point)
_____		*Total score*
		ASSESS level of consciousness
		along a continuum_____
		Alert Drowsy Stupor Coma

TABLE 7–2   Folstein's "Mini-Mental State" *Continued*

INSTRUCTIONS FOR ADMINISTRATION OF MINI-MENTAL STATE EXAMINATIONS

Orientation
(1) Ask for the date. Then ask specifically for parts omitted, e.g, "Can you also tell me what season it is?" 1 point for each correct.

(2) Ask in turn "Can you tell me the name of this hospital?" (town, county, etc.). 1 point for each correct.

Registration
Ask the patient if you may test his memory. Then say the names of 3 unrelated objects, clearly and slowly, about one second for each. After you have said all 3 ask him to repeat them. This first repetition determines his score (0–3) but keep saying them until he can repeat all 3 up to 6 trials. If he does not eventually learn all 3, recall cannot be meaningfully tested.

Attention and Calculation
Ask the patient to begin with 100 and count backwards by 7. Stop after 5 subtractions (93, 86, 79, 72, 65). Score the number of correct answers.

If the patient cannot or will not perform this task, ask him to spell the word "world" backwards. The score is the number of letters in correct order. E.g., dlrow = 5, dlorw = 3.

Recall
Ask the patient if he can recall the 3 words you previously asked him to remember. Score 0–3.

Language
Naming: Show the patient a wrist watch and ask him what it is. Repeat for pencil. Score 0–2.

Repetition: Ask the patient to repeat the sentence after you. Allow only one trial. Score 0 or 1.

3-Stage command: Give the patient a piece of plain blank paper and repeat the command. Score 1 point for each part correctly executed.

Reading: On a blank piece of paper, print the sentence "Close your eyes" in letters large enough for the patient to see clearly. Ask him to read it and do what it says. Score 1 point only if he actually closes his eyes.

Writing: Give the patient a blank piece of paper and ask him to write a sentence for you. Do not dictate a sentence; it is to be written spontaneously. It must contain a subject and verb and be sensible. Correct grammar and punctuation are not necessary.

Copying: On a clean piece of paper, draw intersecting pentagons, each side about 1 in., and ask him to copy it exactly as it is. All 10 angles must be present and 2 must intersect to score 1 point. Tremor and rotation are ignored.

Estimate the patient's level of sensorium along a continuum, from alert on the left to coma on the right.

CHAPTER 8

The Physical Examination of a Geriatric Patient

Grow old along with me!
The best is yet to be,
The last of life, for which the first was made.
Our times are in his hand.
Robert Browning
1812–1889

It is important for the health care provider to recognize that disrobing may be embarrassing for the older patient, especially because examiners are usually much younger than the patients. Modesty must be respected. Make sure that only the area being examined is exposed! Try to make sure that the room is warm; older individuals tend to chill easily. Finally, remember that putting on a robe or gown for a younger patient may not present any difficulty, but for an older patient who may have difficulty in moving, perhaps because of arthritis, it may be a real problem.

The physical examination of the geriatric patient is no different from that of the adult patient. Special attention, however, should be given to the following areas: vital signs; skin; head, eyes, ears, nose, throat, and neck; breasts; chest; cardiovascular system; abdomen; musculoskeletal examination; and neurologic examination.

Assessment of Vital Signs

Assess *blood pressure including orthostatic changes* in pulse and blood pressure (pp. 295–298). Be careful if the patient complains of dizziness or chest discomfort! If the patient becomes orthostatic, have the patient lie down immediately.

Obtain *body temperature*. It is important to recognize that in the geriatric population, a normal temperature is commonly found in patients with severe infections (p. 651).

Obtain accurate *weight* (p. 651).

Skin

Observe the skin for any *malignant changes, pressure sores, evidence of pruritus, and ecchymoses suggestive of falls or abuse.*

Head, Eyes, Ears, Nose, Throat, and Neck

Evaluate the patient for any *evidence of skull trauma* (p. 140).

Palpate the *superficial temporal arteries,* which are located anterosuperior to the tragus (p. 651).

Is *entropion or ectropion* present?

Determine *visual acuity* (p. 159).

Evaluate the *cardinal positions of gaze* to exclude gaze palsies (pp. 162–163). Remember that the ability to gaze upward declines with increasing age.

Perform *funduscopic examination.* Are cataracts present? Examine the retina if the patient has no cataract. Is macular degeneration present (pp. 172–176)?

Evaluate *auditory acuity* (pp. 203–206).

Is *cerumen impacted* in the external canal (pp. 206–207)?

Ask the patient to remove any dentures, if present. *Examine the mouth* for dryness, lesions, condition of teeth, oral ulcers, or malignancies (pp. 230–234).

Examine the *tongue for malignancy* (p. 234).

Auscultate the neck. Are carotid bruits present (pp. 326–327)?

Palpate the *thyroid gland.* Are nodules present? Is the thyroid gland diffusely enlarged (p. 142)?

Breasts

Examine the *breasts for dimpling, discharge, or masses* (pp. 344–351, 651).

Chest

Inspect the *shape of the chest* (pp. 259–260). Is kyphoscoliosis present?

Auscultate the chest (pp. 265–267). Are any adventitious sounds present?

Cardiovascular System

Evaluate the *point of maximum impulse* (p. 304). Is it displaced laterally?

Auscultate the heart in the four main positions (pp. 307–310). Are any murmurs, rubs, or gallops heard (p. 652)?

Are the *peripheral pulses* present (pp. 324–332)? Is there evidence of peripheral vascular disease (p. 652)?

Abdomen

Perform routine *inspection, auscultation, palpation and percussion* (pp. 366–380). Is the bladder enlarged?

Is a *pulsatile abdominal mass* present (p. 327)?

Palpate for *inguinal and femoral hernias* (pp. 410–411).

Is there evidence of *urine leakage* on the undergarments?

Perform a *rectal examination* (pp. 380–386). Examine the *stool* for blood.

In a man, is the *prostate enlarged* (p. 384)?

Musculoskeletal Examination

Perform a *screening musculoskeletal examination* (pp. 463–468). Ask the patient to stand up from a seated position, and observe for any difficulties. Can the patient lift the hands over the head in order to brush his or her hair?

The extremities should be examined for arthritis, impaired range of motion, and deformities. The feet should be inspected carefully for nail care, calluses, deformities, and peripheral pulses.

Neurologic Examination

Evaluate the *mental status* carefully, if not already done (p. 649).

Check *vibration sensation* (p. 652).

Test *deep tendon reflexes* (pp. 529–534, 652).

Evaluate *upper extremity tone* for cogwheeling (pp. 526, 652).

Perform *Romberg's test* (p. 542).

Evaluate *gait* (pp. 542–543).

Any elderly patient with a change in function must be evaluated for dementia, depression, and Parkinson's disease.

SECTION V

The Clinical Evaluation of the Acutely Ill Patient

CHAPTER 9

The Acutely Ill Patient

Ther is no thing more precious here than tyme.*
Saint Bernard
1090–1153

This chapter provides a practical approach to the acutely ill patient. The emphasis is on diagnosis, *not* on therapy. In the assessment of the acutely ill patient, time is critical. Unlike assessment of the stable patient, the evaluation of the acutely ill patient does not involve achieving a specific diagnosis but rather identifying a pathophysiologic abnormality that may appear to be identical for several diagnoses. In the evaluation of the acutely ill patient, always ask yourself, What is the most serious threat to life, and have I ruled it out? Remember also that **your** health is vitally important. Exposure to body substances places you at risk. The minimum isolation precaution for an emergency response is the wearing of latex gloves.

As you approach the apparent victim when you are delivering healthcare in the field and perhaps even in the hospital, always perform a brief evaluation to determine whether you are in a safe environment; if not, dispose yourself and your patient to limit exposure to possible injury. This may be a rare situation, but in circumstances where it is likely that the rescuer may be injured or killed while rendering care, the rescuer should wait until the situation can be made safe. It does not help the patient if the rescuer is injured. For example, the patient trapped in a car that is in a busy traffic lane should **not** be given first aid until safety flares or cones can be placed to prevent secondary accidents.

During the evaluation survey, as you approach the scene of the accident, you should search for other victims who may be hidden from view. During this survey you will also be able to appreciate the mechanism(s) of injury and attempt to memorize the scene for later reconsideration in the emergency department and perhaps as a witness for the injured plaintiff.

The task for the clinician in approaching most, if not all, patients in acute situations is to first ascertain that these patients are not in cardiopulmonary arrest or do not have major perturbations of their vital signs to the point that their continued viability is threatened. The general approach to these acute undefined encounters is to **consider the patient unstable** until you can confirm, through a series of diagnostic steps, that the patient is well enough for you to take the time to perform a more rigorous and complete history and physical examination.

This strategy leads you to rapidly access and move through a series of simple algorithms that are grouped into two major categories termed the *primary* and *secondary surveys*. The ***primary survey*** is a check for conditions that are an immediate threat to

*There is nothing more precious here than time.

the patient's life. This initial assessment should take no longer than 30 seconds. The primary survey is in turn subdivided into a *Cardiopulmonary Resuscitation (CPR) Survey* and a *Key Vital Functions Assessment*. The algorithms for the primary survey are shown in Figures 9–1 and 9–2. The ***secondary survey*** is a check for conditions that could become life-threatening problems if not recognized and attended to. An acutely ill patient is anxious and frightened; a calm and reassuring voice can go a long way toward comforting the patient. It is always easier to care for a more relaxed patient than an anxious one.

The primary and secondary surveys approach is used for both adult and pediatric patients, as well as for medical and injury-related problems. Inherent in the approach is that the treatment process is inextricably integrated into the diagnostic process. For example, if the patient is not breathing, ventilations are begun immediately, before moving on to the next diagnostic step in the algorithm.

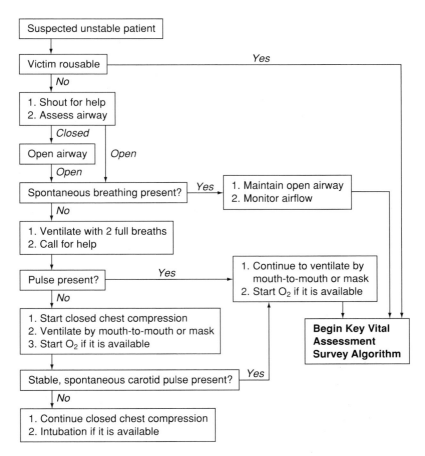

Figure 9–1   Cardiopulmonary Resuscitation (CPR) Survey Algorithm.

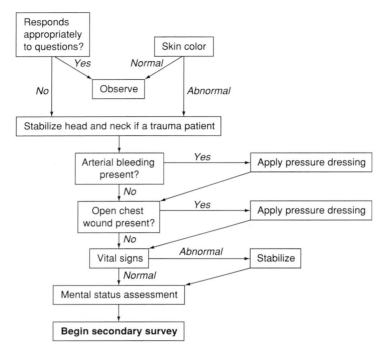

Figure 9–2   Key Vital Functions Assessment Algorithm.

The first task is to recognize an acutely ill patient. An unusual appearance or behavior may be the only signs of a critically ill patient. These include breathing difficulties, clutching the chest or throat, slurring of speech, confusion, unusual odor to the breath, sweating for no apparent reason, or an uncharacteristic skin color (e.g., pale, flushed, or bluish).

PRIMARY SURVEY

CPR Survey

It should not be assumed that any patient who is not obviously interacting with his or her environment is simply sleeping. For the purpose of this approach, the patient is in cardiopulmonary arrest until proven otherwise. As you approach the patient, observe him or her closely, looking for spontaneous breathing or movements. If these are not discernible, access the algorithm as follows:

> *Stimulate the patient by talking loudly to him.*
> *If necessary, shout: ARE YOU OKAY?*

If there is no response, obtain an open **airway** by the chin lift–head tilt maneuver and look, listen, and feel (feel air movement against your cheek) for breathing. To open an unconscious victim's airway, hyperextend the head and lift the chin; place one hand on the forehead and the other behind the occiput and tilt the head backward. This maneuver moves the tongue away from the back of the throat, allowing air to pass around the tongue and into the trachea. **Caution should be exercised in any patient in whom there is a suspected neck injury.** In patients with a suspected neck injury, try to open the airway by lifting the chin without tilting the head backward; grasp the lower teeth and pull the mandible forward. If necessary, tilt the head back very slightly. If a patient is wearing dentures, remove them only if they occlude the airway.

If there is no evidence of spontaneous **breathing**, deliver two full breaths using mouth-to-mouth ventilation. Next, call for help in any way you can without leaving the patient, as your patient is *in extremis*; it is unlikely that you can manage the entire resuscitation by yourself.

Determine whether there is spontaneous **cardiac function** by feeling for a carotid pulse, or in an infant, palpate the precordium for a cardiac impulse. If there is no pulse, begin external chest compression and intersperse it with your ventilations—in other words, begin cardiopulmonary resuscitation.

Key Vital Functions Assessment Survey

Once it has been determined that the patient does not need CPR, or has recovered spontaneous cardiopulmonary activity, you must next ascertain whether key life-sustaining functions are adequate and stable or require augmentation or other supportive measures. In the initial overview of the patient, two observations can save a great deal of time and will help avoid unnecessary or untimely interventions:

1. If the patient's central nervous system is functioning as manifested by the patient's ability to respond appropriately to questions, it is unlikely that the key vital functions are so deranged as to require immediate intervention.
2. If the patient's skin is warm, dry, and of normal color, it is fair to say that there is adequate oxygenation and flow of blood to the periphery.

In shock, peripheral blood flow is shunted centrally. Thus skin changes are early indicators of hypovolemic or cardiogenic (low cardiac output) shock. The key diagnostic signs in the skin that would be associated with these major acute cardiopulmonary derangements include gray, mottled or cyanotic color, cold skin temperature, and markedly sweaty skin. The latter sign, termed *diaphoresis*, is caused by the activation of the sympathetic nervous system by any major threat to homeostasis.

At this point in the process in a patient who possibly has sustained a head injury, it is critical to immobilize the patient's head and neck using boards, tape, and bulky dressing or towels or simply to assign someone to hold the head immobile. Once the evaluation is completed and the imaging studies performed, where necessary the patient can be freed of restriction to movement. Once the patient is immobilized, however, the decision to demobilize should be made carefully.

The next two priorities are the search for, and the management of, arterial bleeding and open chest injuries. Open chest injuries are termed *sucking chest wounds*, as they allow air to enter the pleural space and collapse the underlying lung (pneumothorax). Both arterial bleeding and a sucking chest wound can cause death in a short period, and both are treated by occluding the area with a pressure dressing.

At this point in the algorithm the patient has been stabilized sufficiently to allow signs to be obtained formally. In the field these include the patient's mental status, the respiratory rate and pattern, pulse, blood pressure, and in some circumstances, the body temperature. Mental status can be assessed according to the AVPU system or, as more traditionally categorized, as alert, lethargic, stuporous, or comatose. The *AVPU* mnemonic for level of consciousness is

A Patient is *A*lert
V Patient responds to a *V*erbal stimulus
P Patient responds to a *P*ainful stimulus
U Patient is *U*nresponsive

The blood pressure can be estimated by the pulse wave fullness and by assessing which pulses are palpable. Thus, if the radial pulse at the wrist is palpable, the blood pressure is at least 80 mm Hg systolic. If the radial is impalpable and only the femoral pulse is perceptible, the systolic blood pressure is between 60 and 70 mm Hg. If a vital sign is abnormal, treat the abnormality to bring it back toward normal. Thus, if the patient is breathing spontaneously at a rate of 5 breaths per minute, augment and assist the patient's breathing so that the depth and rate of breathing are normalized. This can be accomplished with interspersed mouth-to-mouth ventilations, with a self-inflating bag-valve-mask device, or with endotracheal intubation and placing the patient on a ventilator. In a similar fashion the blood pressure can be supported by raising the legs and emptying the blood stored in the venous system back into the central circulation. The trauma victim should have a cardiopulmonary examination in this survey as well. Here we are seeking to rule in, or rule out, a tension pneumothorax (shift of the heart away from the tension, increased breath sounds over the side with the tension pneumothorax, distended neck veins, subcutaneous emphysema), cardiac tamponade (distended neck veins, distant heart sounds, hypotension, pulsus paradoxus, normal breath sounds), and chest wall disruption (paradoxical movement of a flail segment).

SECONDARY SURVEY

In the secondary survey you take a history from the patient, the patient's relatives, emergency personnel, or from bystanders. The secondary survey is a systematic method of determining whether other conditions or injuries are present and if they need attention. This survey consists of a rapid interview, a check of the vital signs, and a focused physical examination. Here the mnemonic *AMPLE* can be helpful in gathering pertinent information:

A *A*llergies
M *M*edications currently being taken
P *P*ast medical history
L *L*ast meal
E *E*vents preceding the precipitating event

A critical data element in a trauma patient is the mechanism of injury. Did the patient sustain blunt trauma or was a weapon used causing a penetrating injury? In a vehicular accident, ascertain whether the patient was ejected from the car or was wearing a seat belt and whether others were injured or killed in the accident. In addition, trauma victims must have all their bones and joints, including the rib cage and pelvis and facial bones and skull, palpated and gently compressed to determine if there is a fracture step-off or crepitation and must have stability of structure and function checked as well. A screening neurologic examination is necessary to determine whether there are focal cranial nerve, motor, or sensory findings. Most multisystem trauma patients require a rectal examination to determine the presence of blood and tenderness or upward displacement of the prostate. The latter is a sign of urethral injury.

During the physical examination of an injured patient the patient, if alert, can direct you to the appropriate body areas to be evaluated. The assessment of the patient involves examination of three main regions: the head and neck, the torso, and the extremities. Can the victim move his or her neck? Ask the patient to *slowly* move the neck. Can the shoulders be moved? Ask the patient to take a deep breath in and then blow it out. Does this elicit any pain? Is the patient able to move his or her fingers? Can the arms be bent? Can the patient move his or her toes? Ankles? Can the patient bend his or her legs? If the patient can move all extremities without experiencing pain, slowly help the patient up to a sitting position. If the patient cannot move a body part or can do so only with pain, reassess the airway, breathing, and circulation and get immediate assistance. Continue to observe the patient's level of consciousness, breathing, and skin color.

Head and Neck

Look at the victim's face. Evaluate skin color and temperature. Is there evidence of *raccoon eyes* or *Battle's sign*? A patient with raccoon eyes is shown in Figure 9–3. Periorbital

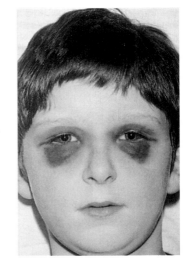

Figure 9–3   Battle's sign or raccoon eyes.

TABLE 9–1   Eye Signs in a Comatose Patient*

Eye Sign	Possible Causes
Pupils reactive, eyes directed straight ahead, normal oculocephalic reflex (OCR)†	Toxic/metabolic
Pinpoint pupils	Narcotic poisoning (OCR intact)
	Pontine or cerebellar hemorrhage (OCR absent)
	Thalamic hemorrhage
	Miotic eye drops
Disconjugate deviation of eyes	Structural brainstem lesion
Conjugate lateral deviation of eyes	Ipsilateral pontine infarction
	Contralateral frontal hemispheric infarction
Unilateral dilated pupil, fixed pupil with no consensual responses	Supratentorial mass lesion
	Impending brain herniation
	Posterior communicating aneurysm
Bilateral midposition pupils, fixed pupils	Midbrain lesion
	Impending brain herniation
Raccoon eyes (periorbital ecchymoses)	Fracture of the base of the skull

*Be aware that the eye signs are difficult to evaluate in patients with artificial lenses, prosthetic eyes, contact lenses, cataracts, or after cataract surgery.
†Doll's eyes: Rotate the head quickly but gently from side to side. In an unconscious patient with an intact brainstem the eyes move conjugately in a direction opposite to the head turning.

ecchymoses, or raccoon eyes, are seen 6 to 12 hours after a fracture of the base of the skull. Battle's sign is ecchymosis behind the ear(s) caused by basilar skull or temporal bone fractures; this sign may take 24 to 36 hours to develop. Palpate the head.

Examine the eyes for pupillary size and responsiveness to light. Are the pupils equal? Are the pupils pinpoint? Is there a unilateral dilated pupil? Are the pupils fixed? Table 9–1 reviews the eye signs in a comatose patient.

Is there a discharge from the ears, nose, or mouth?

Inspect the neck. Is the trachea deviated? Suspect a chest injury, such as a tension pneumothorax, if the trachea is not midline. Palpate the neck for crepitus, which is indicative of air under the skin from a rupture of the lung.

Abdomen

Inspect the abdomen. Is there abdominal distension? Is there evidence of blunt abdominal trauma, such as an ecchymosis, abrasion, or an abdominal wound? *Cullen's sign* is a bluish discoloration around the umbilicus indicative of intraabdominal bleeding or trauma. *Grey Turner's sign*, ecchymotic discoloration around the flanks, is suggestive of retroperitoneal bleeding. Swelling or ecchymosis often occurs late; therefore its presence is extremely important.

Gently and carefully palpate the abdomen, noting any tenderness. If the patient is a woman in the childbearing age, always consider the possibility that she may be pregnant.

Inspect the anus and perineum. Inspect the urethral meatus for blood.

Perform a rectal examination to assess anal sphincter tone, to determine whether blood is present, and to verify that the prostate is in its normal position.

Pelvis

Use the heels of your hands to apply gentle downward pressure on both anterior superior iliac spines and on the symphysis pubis. Tenderness may indicate fracture of the pelvic ring.

Extremities

Inspect and palpate all extremities for evidence of injury. Try to determine whether the patient can move all extremities. Palpate all peripheral pulses.

Back

Inspect the back for obvious signs of injury. This can be done by gently insinuating your hands beneath the back and neck without moving the patient. If this cannot be done, the patient should be gently log rolled onto his or her side. To log roll a patient, you will need at least four assistants: one to control the head and neck, two to role the patient's torso onto its side, and one to cautiously move the lower extremities. Figure 9–4 shows the log roll procedure.

Vital Signs

Reassess vital signs.

The history obtained from the acutely ill medical patient conforms closely to the standard history and physical, but it is abbreviated to allow rapid diagnostic and management decisions to be made. The physical examination of the acutely ill nontrauma patient includes a cardiopulmonary examination and examinations of the abdomen and the peripheral pulses.

THE PEDIATRIC EMERGENCY

When assessing the acutely ill child, always consider the similarities and differences of the pediatric age group versus the adult patient; approach the pediatric emergency

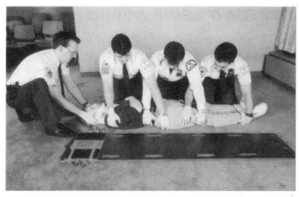

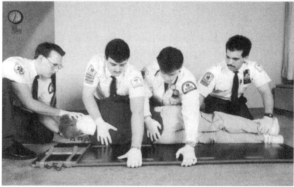

Figure 9–4 Log roll procedure.

1. Apply a cervical spine immobilization device (CSID) and place the patient's arms by his side. Note that one EMT maintains cervical immobilization manually throughout this procedure.
2. Three EMTs can be positioned at the side of the patient at the level of the chest, hips, and lower extremities while the long spine board is positioned on one side of the patient.
3. Check the patient's arm on the side of the EMTs for injury before log rolling the patient and then align the lower extremities.
   Note: The EMT at the lower extremities holds the patient's lower leg and thigh region; the EMT at the hips holds the patient's lower legs and places the other hand on the top of the patient's buttocks; and the EMT at the chest holds the patient's arms against the body and at the level of the lower buttocks.
4. On command from the EMT at the head, all EMTs should rotate the patient toward themselves, keeping the body in alignment.
5. The EMTs then reach across with one hand and pull the board beneath the patient's arm.
6. On command from the EMT at the head, they gently roll the patient onto the board and then roll the board to the ground.
7. Strap the patient's torso and extremities securely to the board and immobilize the head.

From Henry MC, Stapleton ER (eds): EMT Prehospital Care, 2nd ed. Philadelphia, WB Saunders, 1997.

as you would an emergency in an adult but keeping in mind the smaller size of the patient and the difference in the physiologic responses to acute illness and injury. The primary assessment of the child is the same as that of the adult.

The most important life-threatening pediatric emergency is respiratory distress. Respiratory distress in the pediatric patient may arise from a variety of conditions that result from upper or lower airway disease. Common pediatric respiratory problems of the upper airway include croup (laryngotracheobronchitis), epiglottitis, foreign bodies, and bacterial tracheitis. Lower airway obstruction may result from asthma, pneumonia, bronchiolitis, and foreign bodies.

The hallmarks of respiratory distress are tachypnea, nasal flaring, retractions, stridor, cyanosis, head bobbing, prolonged expiration, and grunting. Children with upper airway disease almost always exhibit stridor. In a child with stridor, it is vital to distinguish between croup and epiglottitis; a child with epiglottitis may have a rapid progression to respiratory failure. Fortunately the incidence of epiglottitis has decreased recently, presumably because of the *Haemophilus influenzae* type b (HIB) vaccine. **If epiglottitis is suspected, do not examine the airway without being prepared to intervene in airway stabilization on an emergent basis.** Manipulation of the child's airway can lead to complete airway obstruction. Table 9–2 compares some of the important differences between epiglottitis and croup.

The peak age for foreign body aspiration is between 1 and 2 years. In a child you should consider relief of airway obstruction if

- The child is choking
- The cough becomes ineffective
- Breathing becomes stridorous
- There is loss of consciousness
- The child becomes cyanotic

TABLE 9–2 Differentiation Between Epiglottitis and Croup

Characteristics	Epiglottitis	Croup
Etiology	*H. influenzae* type b	Viral, usually parainfluenza virus
Age of child	Any age (peak 3–7 years)	3 months–3 years
Clinical appearance	Toxic	Not toxic
Season	No seasonal preference	Autumn and winter
Clinical onset	Rapid	Insidious
Upper respiratory tract infection	Rare	Common
Fever	>104° F (40° C)	<103° F (39.4° C)
Sore throat	Severe	Variable
Cough	Not "barking" throughout the day	"Barking" during the night
Drooling	Prominent	None
Stridor	Inspiration	Inspiration and expiration
Position	Sitting forward with neck extended and mouth open	Variable
Epiglottis	Bright red	Normal

Immediately place the infant face down, with the head lower than the torso, on the rescuer's arm, which is placed on his or her thigh. Support the head of the infant by holding his or her jaw. Deliver five forceful back blows with the heel of the hand between the infant's scapulae. Turn the infant on his or her back while holding the head. Place two finger tips on the middle portion of the sternum, one finger breadth below the nipples. Depress the sternum 1 inch (2.5 cm). Repeat this maneuver up to five times. Attempt to remove any visible material from the pharynx. Repeat the back blows and chest thrusts until the object is dislodged.

If the infant becomes unconscious, check the mouth for a foreign body and then perform mouth-to-mouth breathing. Gently tilt the child's head back while placing the fingers of the other hand under the jaw at the chin and lift the chin upward. Seal the child's mouth and nose with your mouth. Deliver two breaths while watching the chest rise. Repeat the back blows and chest thrusts. Have someone call for help.

Dehydration is another important pediatric emergency. The most common causes are vomiting and diarrhea. In a child with mild dehydration (< 5%) there may be only a slight decrease in mucous membrane moisture. In severe dehydration (15%) the following will commonly be found:

- Parched mucous membranes; no tears
- Markedly decreased skin turgor
- Sunken fontanelles
- Tachypnea
- Capillary refill* >2 seconds
- Skin cool and clammy
- Orthostatic hypotension; systolic pressure < 80 mm Hg
- Tachycardia; >130 beats per minute

Intravenous infusion of isotonic fluids should be started immediately in children with severe dehydration.

The secondary assessment as outlined earlier and the AVPU mnemonic are as important for the child as for the adult. Table 9–3 provides a useful reference for CPR.

---

*Capillary refill is an assessment of perfusion. It is the time it takes for a patient's skin color to return to normal after the nailbed has been pressed. The normal refill time is less than 2 seconds.

TABLE 9–3 Cardiopulmonary Resuscitation Reference Chart

	Infant (<1 Year Old)	Child (>1 Year Old)	Adult
If victim has a pulse, give 1 breath every	3 seconds	3 seconds	5–6 seconds
If victim has **no** pulse, locate compression landmark	1 finger breadth below the nipple line	1 finger on sternum	1 finger on sternum
Compressions are performed with	2 or 3 fingers on sternum	Heel of hand on sternum	2 hands stacked with heel of 1 hand on sternum
Rate of compressions per minute	>100	100	80–100
Compression depth (inches)	$\frac{1}{2}$–1	1–1$\frac{1}{2}$	1$\frac{1}{2}$–2
Ratio of compressions to breaths with			
1 rescuer	5:1	5:1	15:2
2 rescuers	5:1	5:1	5:1

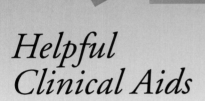

Helpful
Clinical Aids

CHAPTER 10

Helpful Clinical Aids

"Never mind," said Holmes, laughing; "it is my business to know things. Perhaps I have trained myself to see what others overlook. If not, why should you come to consult me?"
Sir Arthur Conan Doyle
1859–1930

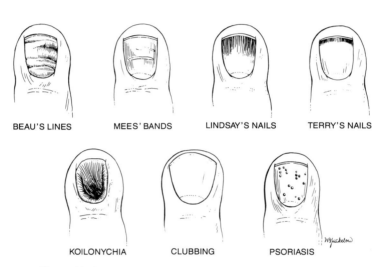

| BEAU'S LINES | MEES' BANDS | LINDSAY'S NAILS | TERRY'S NAILS |

| KOILONYCHIA | CLUBBING | PSORIASIS |

Figure 10–1   Common nail findings associated with medical diseases.

Primary Skin Lesions

1. **Flat, nonpalpable lesions** (Fig. 10–2)
   - *Macule:* Small—up to 1 cm; flat and circumscribed. Examples: freckles, flat nevi, hypopigmentation, petechiae.
   - *Patch:* Larger than 1 cm. Examples: vitiligo, chloasma, mongolian spot, café au lait spot.

2. **Palpable, solid lesions** (Fig. 10–3)
   - *Papule:* Up to 0.5 cm. Examples: mole, lichen planus, wart.
   - *Nodule:* Size 0.5 to 2 cm; often extends deeper into the dermis than does a papule. Examples: xanthoma, fibroma.

154

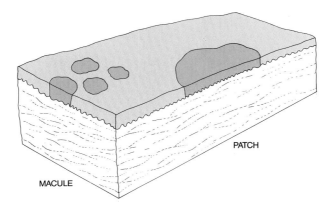

Figure 10–2   Primary lesions (flat, nonpalpable).

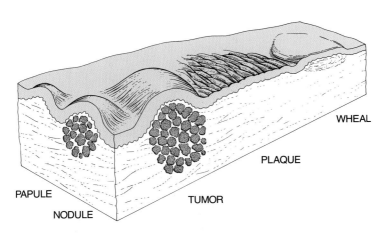

Figure 10–3   Primary lesions (palpable, elevated, solid masses).

- *Tumor:* Larger than 2 cm; may be benign or malignant; may be firm or soft. Examples: lipoma, hemangioma.
- *Plaque:* Elevated flat surface larger than 0.5 cm; plateau-like, disk-shaped lesion. Examples: psoriasis, xanthelasma, lichen planus.
- *Wheal:* Relatively transient, superficial area of local skin edema. Examples: allergic reaction, dermatographism, mosquito bite.

3. **Palpable, fluid-filled lesions** (Fig. 10–4)
   - *Vesicle:* Up to 0.5 cm; contains clear fluid. Examples: herpes simplex, contact dermatitis (e.g., poison ivy), herpes zoster.
   - *Bulla:* Greater than 0.5 cm; filled with clear fluid; thin walled. Examples: burns, contact dermatitis, friction blister, pemphigus.
   - *Pustule:* Filled with pus. Examples: acne, impetigo.

4. **Special primary lesions** (Fig. 10–5)
   - *Comedo:* Example: blackhead.
   - *Burrow:* Example: scabies.
   - *Cyst:* Encapsulated, fluid-filled cavity. Example: sebaceous cyst.
   - *Abscess*
   - *Furuncle*
   - *Carbuncle*
   - *Milia*

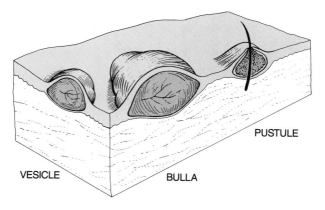

Figure 10–4   Primary lesions (palpable, elevated, fluid-filled masses).

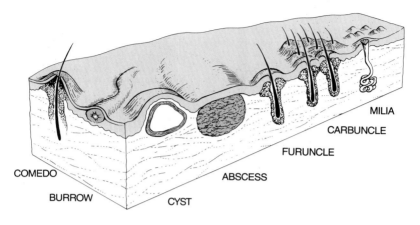

Figure 10–5   Special primary lesions.

Secondary Skin Lesions

1. **Lesions below the skin plane** (Fig. 10–6)
   - *Erosion:* Scooped-out, shallow depression; loss of superficial epidermis that does not bleed or scar. Example: skin after a vesicle has ruptured.
   - *Ulcer:* Deeper depression and loss of tissue that may bleed and scar. Examples: chancre, pressure sore.
   - *Fissure:* Linear crack. Examples: athlete's foot, cheilosis.
   - *Excoriation:* Self-inflicted superficial abrasion. Examples: insect bites, chickenpox, scabies.

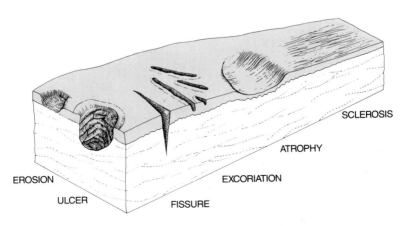

Figure 10–6   Secondary lesions below the skin plane.

- *Atrophy:* thinning of epidermis with depressed loss of tissue. Examples: striae, insulin injections.
- *Sclerosis:* Thickening of skin, producing packed areas of papules.

2. **Lesions above the skin plane** (Fig. 10–7)
    - *Scaling:* Thin flakes of exfoliated epidermis. Examples: psoriasis, eczema, seborrheic dermatitis.
    - *Crusting:* Dried residue of serum, pus, or blood. Examples: scab, weeping eczematous dermatitis.

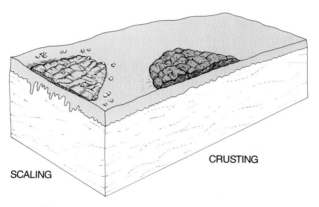

CRUSTING

SCALING

Figure 10–7   Secondary lesions above the skin plane.

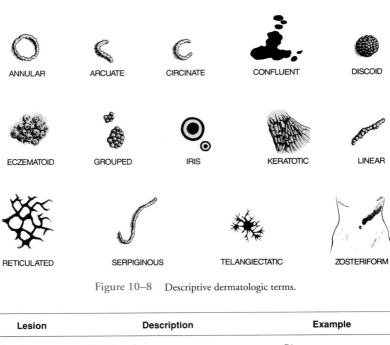

Figure 10–8   Descriptive dermatologic terms.

Lesion	Description	Example
Annular	Ring shaped	Ringworm
Arcuate	Partial rings	Syphilis
Bizarre	Irregular or geographic pattern not related to any underlying anatomic structure	Factitial dermatitis
Circinate	Circular	
Confluent	Lesions run together	Childhood exanthems
Discoid	Disc shaped without central clearing	Lupus erythematosus
Discrete	Lesions remain separate	
Eczematoid	An inflammation with a tendency to vesiculate and crust	Eczema
Generalized	Widespread	
Grouped	Lesions clustered together	Herpes simplex
Iris	Circle within a circle; a bull's-eye lesion	Erythema multiforme (iris)
Keratotic	Horny thickening	Psoriasis
Linear	In lines	Poison ivy dermatitis
Multiform	More than one type of shape or lesion	Erythema multiforme
Papulosquamous	Papules or plaques associated with scaling	Psoriasis
Reticulated	Lace-like network	Oral lichen planus
Serpiginous	Snake-like, creeping	Cutaneous larva migrans
Telangiectatic	Relatively permanent dilatation of the superficial blood vessels	Osler-Weber-Rendu disease
Universal	Entire body involved	Alopecia universalis
Zosteriform*	Linear arrangement along a nerve distribution	Herpes zoster

*Also known as dermatomal.

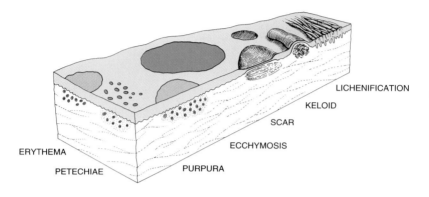

Figure 10–9   Other important dermatologic terms.

Lesion	Description	Example
Erythema	Pink or red blanchable discoloration of the skin secondary to dilatation of blood vessels	
Petechiae	Purplish-red, nonblanchable, pinpoint flat spots caused by intradermal or submucosal hemorrhage	
Purpura	Purple, nonblanchable discoloration of the skin as a result of extravasation of blood	
Ecchymosis	Large purpuric lesions, generally greater than 1 cm	"Black and blue mark"
Scar	Connective tissue replacement following dermal tissue loss	
Alopecia	Loss of hair	
Keloid	Hypertrophied scar tissue	
Lichenification	A thickening and roughening of skin with accentuation of the normal skin lines	

TABLE 10–1 Common Maculopapular Diseases*

	Psoriasis	Pityriasis Rosea	Tinea Versicolor	Seborrheic Dermatitis	Lichen Planus
Color	Dull red, silvery	Pinkish yellow	Reddish brown	Pinkish yellow	Violaceous
Scale	Abundant	Fine, adherent	Fine	Greasy	Shiny, adherent
Induration	1+	0	0	1+	1+
Face lesions	Rarely	Rarely	Occasionally	Common	Rarely
Oral lesions	0	0	0	0	2+
Nail lesions	4+	0	0	0	Rarely

*See Figures 6–12, p. 102; 6–44 and 6–45, p. 115; 6–51, 116; 6–58, p. 119; and 6–77 and 6–78, p. 127, in *Textbook of Physical Diagnosis.*
0, rarely seen; 1+, occasionally seen; 2+, frequently seen; 4+, nearly always associated.

TABLE 10–2 Common Eczematous Diseases*

	Contact Dermatitis	Atopic Dermatitis	Neurodermatitis	Stasis Dermatitis
History	Acute, localized to specific area	History in patient or family member of asthma, hay fever, or eczema	Chronic, in same areas, associated with anxiety	Varicosities, history of thrombophlebitis or cellulitis
Location	Areas of exposure to allergen	Eyelids, groin, flexural areas	Head, lower legs, arms	Lower legs

*See Figures 6–42, p. 114; 6–83, p. 129; and 6–84, p. 130, in *Textbook of Physical Diagnosis.*

TABLE 10–3 Vesiculobullous Diseases*

	Pemphigus Vulgaris	Dermatitis Herpetiformis	Epidermolysis Bullosa†	Bullous Pemphigoid
Age of patient	40–60	Children or adults	Infants or children	60–70
Initial site	Oral mucosa	Scalp, trunk	Extremities	Extremities
Lesions	Normal skin at margins	Erythematous base	Bullae produced by trauma	Normal skin at margins
Sites	Mouth, abdomen, scalp, groin	Knees, sacrum, back, elbows	Hands, knees, elbows, mouth, toes	Trunk, extremities
Groupings	0	4+	1+	0
Weight loss	Marked	None	None	Minimal
Duration	1 or more years	Several years	Normal lifetime	Months to years
Pruritus	0	4+	0	±
Oral pain	4+	0	±	±
Palms/soles involved	No	No	Yes	Yes
Typical lesions	Flaccid bulla	Grouped vesicles	Flaccid vesicles	Tense bulla

*See Figures 6–81 and 6–82, p. 129, in *Textbook of Physical Diagnosis.*
†Refers not to a single disorder but to a group of inherited diseases.
0, rarely seen; 1+, occasionally seen; 4+, nearly always associated; ±, sometimes present.

TABLE 10–4   Common Benign Tumors by Color

Color	Benign Tumor
Skin color	Warts (see Fig. 6–24, p. 108)* Cysts Keloids (see Fig. 6–80, p. 128)* Nevi
Pink or red	Hemangiomas (see Fig. 22–7, p. 600)* Keloids
Brown	Seborrheic keratoses (see Fig. 6–79, p. 127)* Nevi Lentigines Dermatofibromas
Tannish yellow	Xanthomata (see Fig. 12–12, p. 292)* Xanthelasma (see Fig. 12–17, p. 294)* Warts Keloids
Dark blue or black	Seborrheic keratoses Hemangiomas Blue nevi Dermatofibromas

*In *Textbook of Physical Diagnosis.*

TABLE 10–5   Symptoms of Hyperthyroidism

Organ System	Symptom
General	Preference for the cold Weight loss with good appetite
Eyes	Prominence of eyeballs* Puffiness of eyelids Double vision Decreased motility
Neck	Goiter
Cardiac	Palpitations Peripheral edema†
Gastrointestinal	Increased bowel movements
Genitourinary	Polyuria Decreased fertility
Neuromuscular	Fatigue Weakness Tremulousness
Emotional	Nervousness Irritability
Dermatologic	Hair thinning Increased perspiration Change in skin texture Change in pigmentation

*Appears to be due to mucopolysaccharide deposition behind the orbit.
†Appears to be due to excessive mucopolysaccharide deposition under the skin, especially in the legs.

TABLE 10–6   Characteristics of Benign and Malignant Thyroid Nodules

Characteristic	Benign Nodule	Malignant Nodule
Age at onset	Adult	Adult
Gender	Female	Male
Patient history	Symptoms present	Previous x-ray treatment to head or neck
Family history	Benign thyroid diseases	None
Speed of enlargement	Slow	Rapid
Change in voice	Absent	Present
Number of nodules	More than one	One
Lymph nodes	Absent	Present
Remainder of thyroid	Abnormal	Normal

TABLE 10–7   Symptoms and Signs of Hypothyroidism

System	Symptom	Sign
General	Weight gain with regular diet Chilly while others are warm	Obesity
Gastrointestinal	Constipation	Enlarged tongue
Cardiovascular	Fatigue	Hypotension Bradycardia
Nervous	Speech disorders Short attention span Tremor	Hyporeflexia Defective abstract reasoning Spasticity Tremor Depressed affect
Musculoskeletal	Lethargy Thickened, dry skin Hair loss Brittle nails Leg cramps Puffy eyelids Puffy cheeks	Hypotonia Puffy facies
Reproductive	Heavier menses Decreased fertility	

TABLE 10–8   Actions and Innervations of the Extraocular Muscles*

Muscle	Action	Cranial Nerve Innervation
Medial rectus	Adduction (eye moves nasally)	Oculomotor (III)
Lateral rectus	Abduction (eye moves temporally [away from the nose])	Abducens (VI)
Inferior rectus	Depression (eye moves down) Extorsion (the 12 o'clock position on the cornea rotates temporally) Adduction	Oculomotor (III)
Superior rectus	Elevation (eye moves up) Intorsion (the 12 o'clock position on the cornea rotates nasally) Adduction	Oculomotor (III)
Superior oblique	Depression Intorsion Abduction	Trochlear (IV)
Inferior oblique	Elevation Extorsion Abduction	Oculomotor (III)

*Remember "LR_6SO_4." This mnemonic states that the lateral rectus (LR) muscle is innervated by the sixth cranial nerve and the superior oblique (SO) muscle is innervated by the fourth cranial nerve. All the other muscles are innervated by the third cranial nerve.

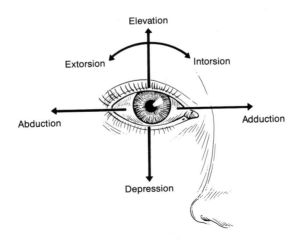

Figure 10–10   Extraocular movements.

TABLE 10–9   Common Visual Eye Symptoms and Disease States

Visual Symptom	Possible Causes
Loss of vision	Optic neuritis Detached retina Retinal hemorrhage Central retinal vascular occlusion Central nervous system disease
Spots	No pathologic significance*
Flashes	Migrane Retinal detachment Posterior vitreous detachment
Loss of visual field or presence of shadows or curtains	Retinal detachment Retinal hemorrhage
Glare, photophobia	Iritis (inflammation of the iris) Meningitis (inflammation of the meninges)
Distortion of vision	Retinal detachment Macular edema
Difficulty seeing in dim light	Myopia Vitamin A deficiency Retinal degeneration
Colored haloes around lights	Acute narrow angle glaucoma Opacities in lens or cornea
Colored vision changes	Cataracts Drugs (digitalis increases yellow vision)
Double vision	Extraocular muscle paresis or paralysis

*May precede a retinal detachment or may be associated with ingestion of fertility drugs.

TABLE 10–10 Common Nonvisual, Painful Eye Symptoms and Disease States

Nonvisual, Painful Symptom	Possible Causes
Foreign body sensation	Foreign body Corneal abrasion
Burning	Uncorrected refractive error Conjunctivitis Sjögren's syndrome
Throbbing, aching	Acute iritis (inflammation of the iris) Sinusitis (inflammation of the sinuses)
Tenderness	Eyelid inflammations Conjunctivitis Iritis
Headache	Refractive errors Migraine Sinusitis
Drawing sensation	Uncorrected refractive errors

TABLE 10–11 Common Nonvisual, Painless Eye Symptoms and Disease States

Nonvisual, Painless Symptom	Possible Causes
Itching	Dry eyes Eye fatigue Allergies
Tearing	Emotional states Hypersecretion of tears Blockage of drainage
Dryness	Sjögren's syndrome Decreased secretion as a result of aging
Sandiness, grittiness	Conjunctivitis
Fullness of eyes	Proptosis (bulging of the eyeball) Aging changes in the lids
Twitching	Fibrillation of orbicularis oculi
Eyelid heaviness	Fatigue Eyelid edema
Dizziness	Refractive error Cerebellar disease Vestibular disease
Excessive blinking	Local irritation Facial tic
Eyelids sticking together	Inflammatory disease of eyelids or conjunctivae

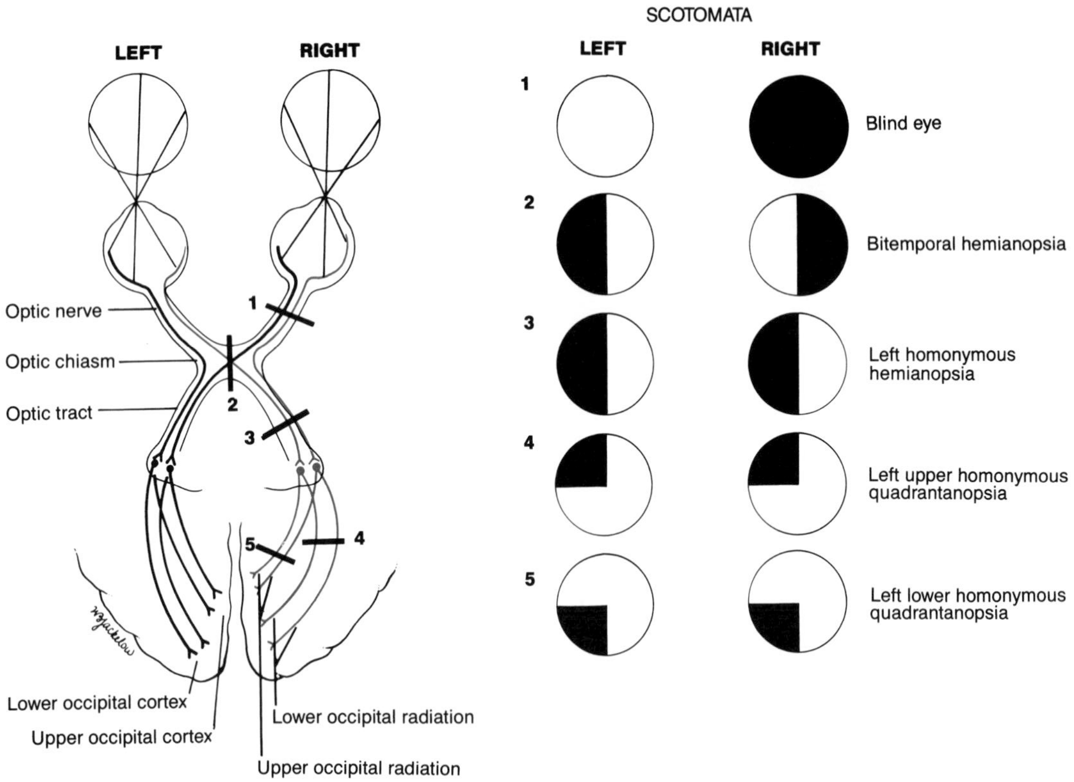

Figure 10–11 Visual field defects.

SCOTOMATA

LEFT | RIGHT

1. Blind eye
2. Bitemporal hemianopsia
3. Left homonymous hemianopsia
4. Left upper homonymous quadrantanopsia
5. Left lower homonymous quadrantanopsia

LEFT | RIGHT

Optic nerve
Optic chiasm
Optic tract
Lower occipital cortex
Upper occipital cortex
Lower occipital radiation
Upper occipital radiation

TABLE 10–12   Differentiation of Whitish Lesions of the Fundus

	Cotton-Wool Spots*	Fatty Exudates†	Drusen‡	Chorioretinitis‖
Etiology§	Hypertension Diabetic retinopathy Acquired immunodeficiency syndrome (AIDS) Lupus erythematosus Dermatomyositis Papilledema	Diabetes mellitus Retinal venous occlusion Hypertensive retinopathy	Can be normal with aging	Toxoplasmosis Sarcoidosis Cytomegalovirus
Border	Fuzzy	Well defined	Well defined, nonpigmented	Often large with ragged edge, heavily pigmented
Shape	Irregular	Small, irregular	Round, well circumscribed	Extremely variable
Patterns	Variable	Often clustered in circles or stars	Variable; symmetric in both eyes	Variable
Comments	Caused by an ischemic infarct of the nerve fiber layer of the retina; obscures retinal blood vessels; usually several in number	In deep retinal layer	Often confused with fatty exudates; deep to retinal blood vessels	Acute with white exudate; healed lesion with pigmented scar (toxoplasmosis)

*See Figures 10–16 to 10–19.
†Also known as "edema residues."
‡Also known as "colloid bodies." See Figure 8–45, p. 183, in *Textbook of Physical Diagnosis.*
§The diseases noted do not comprise a complete etiologic list. Only the most common are indicated.
‖See Figures 8–48 and 8–49, p. 184, and 8–50 to 8–52, p. 185, in *Textbook of Physical Diagnosis.*

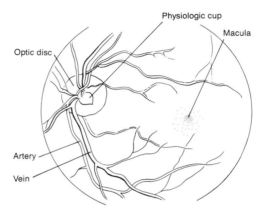

Figure 10–12   Schematic showing the landmarks of the retina of the left eye.

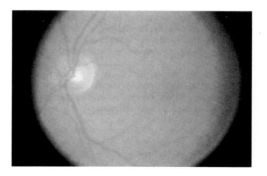

Figure 10–13   Retina: normal.

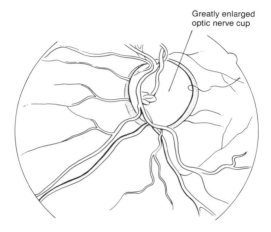

Greatly enlarged
optic nerve cup

Figure 10–14 Labeled schematic of Figure 10–15 , showing glaucomatous cupping of the optic nerve head. The cup-to-disc ratio is approximately 85%.

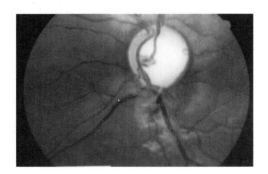

Figure 10–15 Retina: glaucomatous cupping.

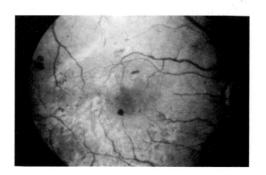

Figure 10–16   Retina: diabetes.

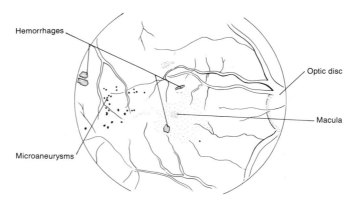

Figure 10–17   Labeled schematic of Figure 10–16, showing the retinal findings in the right eye in a patient with diabetes. Note the microaneurysms at the macula.

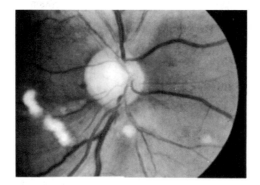

Figure 10–18   Retina: hypertension.

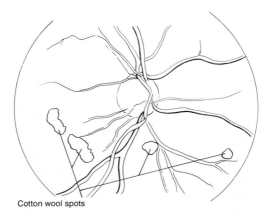

Cotton wool spots

Figure 10–19   Labeled schematic of Figure 10–18, showing the retinal changes in a patient with long-standing hypertension. Note the so-called cotton-wool spots.

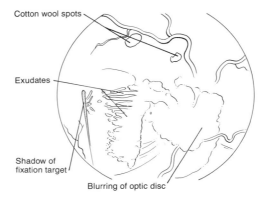

Figure 10–20 Labeled schematic of Figure 10–21, showing the retinal changes in chronic papilledema. Note the marked blurring of the right optic disc, the cotton-wool spots, and the exudates. The dark line at the macula is a shadow of the target at which the patient was asked to look.

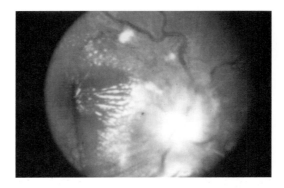

Figure 10–21 Retina: chronic papilledema.

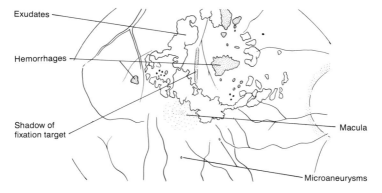

Exudates

Hemorrhages

Shadow of
fixation target

Macula

Microaneurysms

Figure 10–22   Labeled schematic of Figure 10–23, showing the retinal changes of severe diabetes, called *circinate retinopathy*, which is a ring of exudates around the macula. This is the retina of the right eye.

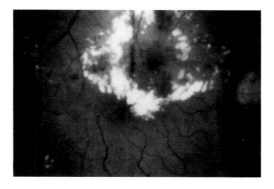

Figure 10–23   Retina: circinate retinopathy.

TABLE 10–13 Differential Diagnosis of the Red Eye*

Presentation	Acute Conjunctivitis†	Acute Iritis‡
History	Sudden onset Exposure to conjunctivitis	Fairly sudden onset Often recurrent
Vision	Normal	Impaired if untreated
Pain	Gritty feeling	Moderate
Bilaterality	Frequent	Occasional
Vomiting	Absent	Absent
Cornea	Clear (epidemic keratoconjunctivitis has corneal deposits)	Variable
Pupil	Normal, reactive	Sluggishly reactive Sometimes irregular in shape
Iris	Normal	Normal‖
Ocular discharge	Mucopurulent or watery	Watery
Systemic effect	None	Few
Prognosis	Self-limited	Poor if untreated

*See Figure 8–37, p. 178, in *Textbook of Physical Diagnosis.*
†Can be viral, bacterial, or allergic.
‡See Figure 8–26, p. 170, in *Textbook of Physical Diagnosis.*
§Seeing "rainbows" can be an early symptom during an acute attack.
‖The ophthalmologist can detect abnormalities with a slit lamp.

Narrow Angle Glaucoma	Corneal Abrasion

Rapid onset
Sometimes history of previous
  attack
Highest incidence among Jews,
  Swedes, and the Inuit
  (Eskimos)
	Trauma
	Pain

Rapidly lost if untreated§	Can be affected if central
Severe	Exquisite
Occasional	Usually unilateral
Common	Absent
"Steamy" (like looking through a steamy window)	Irregular light reflex
Partially dilated, oval, nonreactive	Normal, reactive

Difficult to see, owing to
  corneal edema
	Shadow of corneal defect
	  may be projected on
	  the iris with penlight

Watery	Watery or mucopurulent
Many	None
Poor if untreated	Good if not infected

TABLE 10–14   Differentiation of Blurred Disc Margins

Presentation	Papilledema*	Papillitis†
Visual acuity	Normal	Decreased
Venous pulsations	Absent	Variable
Pain	Headache	Eye movement pain
Light reaction	Present	Marcus Gunn¶
Hemorrhage	Present	Present
Visual fields	Enlarged blindspot	Central scotoma
Laterality	Bilateral	Unilateral

*Edema of the optic disc resulting from increased intracranial pressure. See Figures 10–20 and 10–21.
†Inflammation of the optic disc.
‡See Figure 8–44, p. 182, in *Textbook of Physical Diagnosis.*
§Myelination of the optic nerve ends at the optic disc. When it continues into the retina, white, flamed-shaped areas obscure the disc margins. See Figure 8–34, p. 175, in *Textbook of Physical Diagnosis.*
¶See *Textbook of Physical Diagnosis*, p. 164.

TABLE 10–15   Differentiation of Common Macular Lesions

	Macular Degeneration*
Appearance	Pigmentary mottling, often with hemorrhage
Etiology	

*Often bilateral in the aged.
†See Figure 8–47, p. 183, in *Textbook of Physical Diagnosis.*
‡See Figures 10–22 and 10–23.

Drusen‡	Myelinated Nerve Fibers§	Central Retinal Vein Occlusion‖
Normal	Normal	Decreased
Present	Present	Generally absent
No	No	No
Present	Present	Present
Uncommon	No	Marked
Enlarged blindspot	Scotomata correspond to areas of myelination	Variable
Bilateral	Seldom bilateral	Unilateral

Macular Star†	Circinate Retinopathy‡
Whitish exudate that radiates around macula	Broken ring–shaped whitish exudate around macula
Hypertension	Diabetes
Papilledema	Central retinal vein occlusion
Papillitis	
Central retinal vein occlusion	

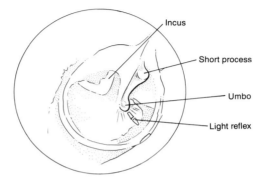

Incus

Short process

Umbo

Light reflex

Figure 10–24   Labeled schematic of Figure 10–25, showing a normal right tympanic membrane.

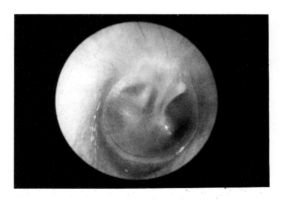

Figure 10–25   Tympanic membrane: normal.

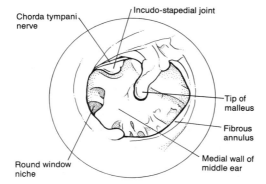

Chorda tympani
nerve

Incudo-stapedial joint

Tip of
malleus

Fibrous
annulus

Medial wall of
middle ear

Round window
niche

Figure 10–26   Labeled schematic of Figure 10–27, showing a central perforation of the right tympanic membrane.

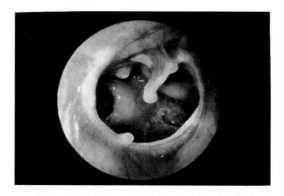

Figure 10–27   Perforated tympanic membrane.

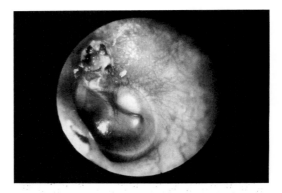

Figure 10–28   Cholesteatoma. Note the injection of the distal external canal.

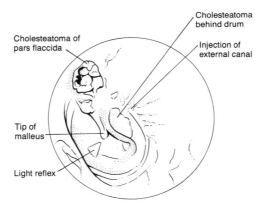

Figure 10–29   Labeled schematic of Figure 10–28, showing a cholesteatoma of the left ear that resulted from a marginal perforation of the tympanic membrane.

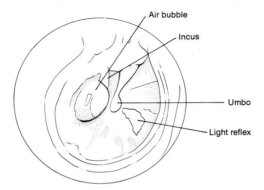

Figure 10–30   Labeled schematic of Figure 10–31, showing serous otitis media of the right ear. Note the air bubble in the middle ear behind the tympanic membrane.

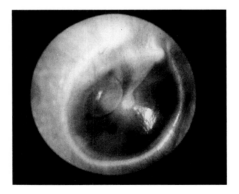

Figure 10–31   Tympanic membrane: serous otitis media.

TABLE 10–16   Comparative Features of Conductive and Sensorineural Hearing Loss

	Conductive Hearing Loss	Sensorineural Hearing Loss
Pathology	External canal Middle ear	Cochlea Cochlear nerve Brain stem
Loudness of speech	Softer than normal	Louder than normal
External canal	May be abnormal	Normal
Tympanic membrane	Usually abnormal	Normal
Rinne test	Negative	Positive
Weber test	Heard on "deaf" side	Heard on better side (only in severe unilateral loss)

TABLE 10–17   Differentiation of Acute External Otitis from Acute Otitis Media

Signs and Symptoms	Acute External Otitis	Acute Otitis Media
Pressure on tragus	Painful	No pain
Lymphadenopathy	Frequent	Absent
External canal	Edematous	Normal
Season	Summer	Winter
Tympanic membrane	Normal	Fluid behind drum, possibly perforated
Fever	Yes	Yes
Hearing loss	Slight or normal	Decreased

TABLE 10–18 Symptoms and Signs of Oral Lesions

Lesion	Symptoms	Signs	Other Information
Aphthous ulcer (canker sore) (see Fig. 10–37, p. 239)	Painful, recurrent white sore with red border on lips, inner side of cheeks, tip and sides of tongue, or palate	Single lesion 0.5–2 cm in diameter that first is maculopapular but then ulcerates and has an area of erythema at its border; lesions usually only on movable mucosal areas	60% of population have periodic canker sores lasting up to 2 weeks; etiology is unknown
Herpetic ulcer (cold sore; fever blister) (see Figs. 10–8, 10–44, p. 242)*	Painful, recurrent sores on the lips	Multiple papules, vesicles or ulcers on the mucocutaneous junction, hard palate, or gingivae; as the bullae break, crusting occurs	*Primary* herpetic infection in children under 16 months of age; multiple lesions in clusters on fixed mucous membranes; small, discrete, whitish vesicles before ulceration; ulcers about 1 mm in diameter, which may coalesce; tender lymphadenopathy, fever, and malaise present; lip lesions represent the *recurrent* form, common in adults; self-limited illness, 1–2 weeks, in both the primary and recurrent forms
Chancre	Painful sore on lips or tongue lasting 2 weeks to 3 months	Single ulcerated lesion with indurated border; lesion without central necrotic material; tender lymphadenitis may be present	

Continued on following page.

AIDS = acquired immunodeficiency syndrome.
*In *Textbook of Physical Diagnosis.*

TABLE 10–18 Symptoms and Signs of Oral Lesions *Continued*

Lesion	Symptoms	Signs	Other Information
Squamous cell carcinoma (see Figs. 10–40, 10–42, and 10–43, p. 241)*	Ulcerated sore of the lips, floor of the mouth, or tongue (especially lateral borders)	Single indurated lesion with indurated and raised border; often in an area of leukoplakia; absence of necrotic material in crater; base often erythematous; speech alterations may result if lesion is large; painless lymphadenopathy may be present in neck; evidence of distant metastasis may be present	Frequently in alcoholics or smokers
Erythema multiforme	Sudden onset of multiple burning ulcers in mouth or on lips	Hemorrhagic areas of ulceration with erythematous bases often with pseudomembrane; lesions start as bullae; skin involvement common (target lesions)	Many precipitating factors include drug reactions, viruses, endocrine changes, and an underlying malignancy; most common in winter and spring in young adults; frequently recurring
Denture hyperplasia	Painless excess tissue at border of denture	Spongy, redundant, often erythematous tissue with impression of edge of denture; frequently seen on anterior maxillary mucosa	
Candidiasis (moniliasis; thrush) (see Figs. 10–25, p. 234, and 10–30, p. 236)*	Burning areas of tongue, inside of cheek, or throat	Whitish pseudomembrane, resembling milk curd, that can be peeled off, leaving a raw, erythematous area that may bleed	Often seen in individuals who are chronically debilitated, patients who are immunosuppressed, or patients receiving long-term antibiotic therapy; commonly seen in persons with AIDS
Erythroplakia (see Figs. 10–18, p. 231, and 10–33, p. 236)*	Painless red area on inside of cheek, tongue, or floor of mouth	Granular, erythematous papules that bleed	High malignant potential

186

Lesion	Symptoms	Clinical Description	Notes
Leukoplakia (see Figs. 10–14, p. 230, 10–15, p. 231, and 10–26, p. 234)*	Painless white area on inside of cheek, tongue, lower lip, or floor of mouth	Hyperkeratinized, whitish lesion that cannot be scraped off; looks similar to flaking white paint; often speckled with reddish areas; associated adenopathy may indicate malignant changes of lesion	Patients are usually men over the age of 40; linked to smoking, AIDS, alcoholism, and chewing tobacco
Lipoma (see Fig. 10–23, p. 233)*	Slow growing, painless mass on inner surface of cheek	Yellowish, nontender, soft mass; freely mobile	
Lichen planus (see Fig. 10–13, p. 230)*	Usually no symptoms; erosive form causes painful, burning sores of inner side of cheeks or tongue	White lesions on buccal mucosa bilaterally in the form of reticulated papules in lacelike pattern; erosive form appears as hemorrhagic, ulcerated lesion with possible white areas or bullae; pseudomembrane may be present over lesion	Nonerosive form is the most common cause of white lesions in the mouth; skin involvement in 10–35% of patients; more frequently seen in patients with emotional stress
Traumatic ulcer	Pain in an area of a sore; short duration (1–2 weeks)	Single lesion with raised erythema at its border; center often with necrotic debris; occasionally purulent; mild lymphadenitis may be present	Patient can frequently relate the cause (e.g., biting cheek while eating)
Mucocele (see Fig. 10–11, p. 230)*	Intermittent, painless swelling of the lower lip or inside of cheek; slightly bluish; occasionally ruptures	Dome-shaped, 1–2 cm in diameter, freely mobile cystic lesion	May be related to trauma or inflammation
Hairy tongue (see Fig. 10–24B, p. 233)*	Gagging sensation associated with "hairy" sensation of tongue; large, blackish, painless lesion on top of tongue	Elongation of filiform papillae on the dorsum of tongue with a change in their color to almost black	History of excessive antibiotic use, excessive use of mouth-wash, poor oral hygiene, smoking, or alcohol use is common
Fordyce's spots (see Fig. 10–16, p. 231)*	None	Clusters of small, yellowish, raised lesions best seen on the buccal mucosa opposite the molar teeth	Common in older individuals; they are normal, hyperplastic sebaceous glands

TABLE 10–19　Tactile Fremitus

Increased	Decreased
Pneumonia Atelectasis (incomplete expansion of lung tissue)	Unilateral 　Pneumothorax 　Pleural effusion 　Bronchial obstruction Bilateral 　Chronic obstructive lung disease 　Chest wall thickening (muscle, fat)

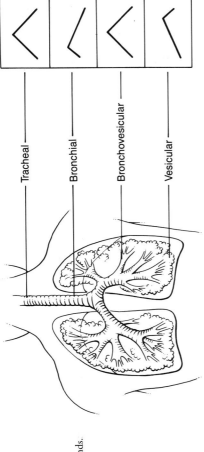

Figure 10–32   Characteristics of breath sounds.

INSPIRATION
EXPIRATION

Tracheal

Bronchial

Bronchovesicular

Vesicular

Characteristic	Tracheal	Bronchial	Bronchovesicular	Vesicular
Intensity	Very loud	Loud	Moderate	Soft
Pitch	Very high	High	Moderate	Low
I:E Ratio*	1:1	1:3	1:1	3:1
Description	Harsh	Tubular	Rustling, but tubular	Gentle rustling
Normal locations	Extrathoracic trachea	Manubrium	Over mainstem bronchi	Most of peripheral lung

*Ratio of duration of inspiration to expiration.

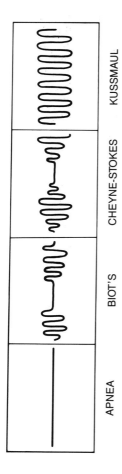

APNEA BIOT'S CHEYNE-STOKES KUSSMAUL

Figure 10–33 Patterns of abnormal breathing.

Pattern	Characteristic	Etiology
Apnea	Absence of breathing	Cardiac arrest
Biot's	Irregular breathing with long periods of apnea	Increased intracranial pressure Drug-induced respiratory depression Brain damage (usually at the medullary level)
Cheyne-Stokes	Irregular breathing with intermittent periods of increased and decreased rates and depths of breaths alternating with periods of apnea	Drug-induced respiratory depression Congestive heart failure Brain damage (usually at the cerebral level)
Kussmaul's	Fast and deep	Metabolic acidosis

TABLE 10–20 Differentiation of Common Pulmonary Conditions

Condition	Vital Signs	Inspection	Palpation	Percussion	Auscultation
Asthma*	Tachypnea; tachycardia	Dyspnea; use of accessory muscles; possible cyanosis; hyperinflation	Often normal; decreased fremitus	Often normal; hyperresonant; low diaphragms	Prolonged expiration; wheezes; decreased lung sounds
Emphysema	Stable	Increased anteroposterior diameter; use of accessory muscles; thin individual	Decreased tactile fremitus	Increased resonance; decreased excursion of diaphragm	Decreased lung sounds; decreased vocal fremitus
Chronic bronchitis	Tachycardia	Possible cyanosis; short, stocky individual	Often normal	Often normal	Early crackles
Pneumonia	Tachycardia; fever; tachypnea	Possible cyanosis; possible splinting on affected side	Increased tactile fremitus	Dull	Late crackles; bronchial breath sounds†

Continued on following page.

*Often the physical findings in asthma are not reliable in predicting its severity.
†Bronchophony, pectoriloquy, and egophony are also often present.

TABLE 10–20 Differentiation of Common Pulmonary Conditions _Continued_

Condition	Vital Signs	Inspection	Palpation	Percussion	Auscultation
Pulmonary embolism	Tachycardia; tachypnea	Often normal	Usually normal	Usually normal	Usually normal
Pulmonary edema	Tachycardia; tachypnea	Possible signs of elevated right heart pressures‡	Often normal	Often normal	Early crackles; wheezes
Pneumothorax	Tachypnea; tachycardia	Often normal; lag on affected side	Absent fremitus; trachea may be shifted to other side	Hyperresonant	Absent breath sounds
Pleural effusion	Tachypnea; tachycardia	Often normal; lag on affected side	Decreased fremitus; trachea shifted to other side	Dullness	Absent breath sounds
Atelectasis	Tachypnea	Often normal; lag on affected side	Decreased fremitus; trachea shifted to other side	Dullness	Absent breath sounds
Adult respiratory distress syndrome (ARDS)	Tachycardia; tachypnea	Use of accessory muscles; cyanosis	Usually normal	Often normal	Normal initially; crackles and decreased lung sounds, late

‡Elevated jugular venous distention, pedal edema, hepatomegaly.

TABLE 10–21   Characteristics of Chest Pain*

	Angina	Not Angina
Location	Retrosternal, diffuse	Left inframammary, localized
Radiation	Left arm, jaw, back	Right arm
Description	"Aching," "dull," "pressing," "squeezing," "vicelike"	"Sharp," "shooting," "cutting"
Intensity	Mild to severe	Excruciating
Duration	Minutes	Seconds, hours, days
Precipitated by	Effort, emotion, eating, cold	Respiration, posture, motion
Relieved by	Rest, nitroglycerin	Nonspecific

*Angina and other chest pain may present in a variety of ways. The characteristics listed here are the common presentations. This list, however, is not absolute. This list should only be used as a guide.

TABLE 10–22   Differentiation of Jugular and Carotid Waveforms

	Internal Jugular Pulse	Carotid Pulse
Palpation	Not palpable	Palpable
Waveforms	Multiform: 2 or 3 components	Single
Quality	Soft, undulating	Vigorous
Pressure*	Waveforms obliterated	No effect
Inspiration	Decreased height of waveforms	No effect
Sitting up	Decreased height of waveforms	No effect
Valsalva maneuver	Increased height of waveforms	No effect

*Light pressure on the vessel above the sternal end of clavicle.

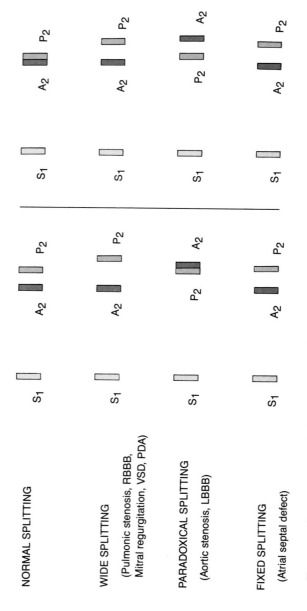

Figure 10–34 Abnormalities of splitting of the second heart sound. (RBBB = right bundle-branch block; VSD = ventricular septal defect; PDA = patent ductus arteriosus; LBBB = left bundle-branch block.)

Type	Description	Cause
Anacrotic	Small, slow rising, delayed pulse with a notch or shoulder on the ascending limb	Aortic stenosis
Waterhammer	Rapid and sudden systolic expansion	Aortic regurgitation
Bisferiens	Double-peaked pulse with a midsystolic dip	Aortic regurgitation Combined aortic stenosis and aortic regurgitation Idiopathic hypertrophic subaortic stenosis (IHSS)
Alternans	Alternating amplitude of pulse pressure	Congestive heart failure
Paradoxical (marked)	Detected by blood pressure assessment. An exaggerated drop in systolic blood pressure during inspiration	Tamponade Constrictive pericarditis Chronic obstructive lung disease

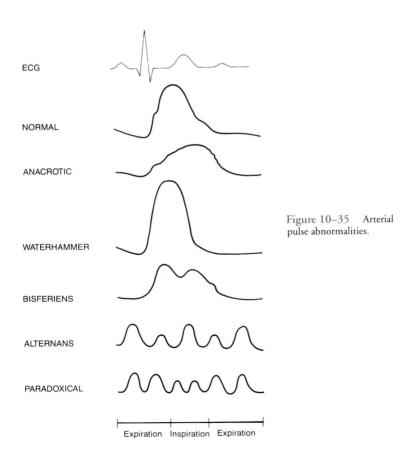

Figure 10–35   Arterial pulse abnormalities.

ECG

NORMAL

ANACROTIC

WATERHAMMER

BISFERIENS

ALTERNANS

PARADOXICAL

Expiration   Inspiration   Expiration

	Aortic Stenosis	Mitral Regurgitation
Location	Aortic area	Apex
Radiation	Neck	Axilla
Shape	Diamond	Holosystolic
Pitch	Medium	High
Quality	Harsh	Blowing
Associated signs	Decreased A_2	Decreased S_1
	Ejection click	S_3
	S_4	Laterally displaced diffuse PMI
	Narrow pulse pressure	
	Slow rising and delayed pulse	

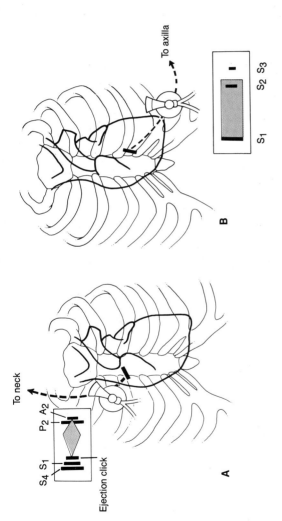

Figure 10–36   Systolic murmurs. *A,* Pathophysiology of aortic stenosis. Note the paradoxical splitting of the second heart sound (S_2), the S_4, and the ejection click. *B,* Mitral regurgitation. Notice that the murmur ends after S_2, and note the presence of the S_3. (PMI = point of maximum impulse.)

	Mitral Stenosis	Aortic Regurgitation
Location	Apex	Aortic area
Radiation	No	No
Shape	Decrescendo	Decrescendo
Pitch	Low	High
Quality	Rumbling	Blowing
Associated signs	Increased S₁	S₃
	Opening snap	Laterally displaced PMI
	RV rock§	Wide pulse pressure*
	Presystolic accentuation	Bounding pulses
		Austin Flint murmur†
		Systolic ejection murmur‡

*The wide pulse pressure is the cause of the many physical signs of aortic regurgitation: Quincke's pulse, de Musset's sign, Duroziez' sign, Corrigan's pulse, etc.
†An apical diastolic murmur heard in association with aortic regurgitation mimicking mitral stenosis.
‡A flow murmur across a valve that is relatively narrow for the increased blood volume as a result of aortic regurgitation. It is relatively stenotic and need not be anatomically stenotic, as in true aortic stenosis.
§Right ventricular impulse at lower left sternal border.

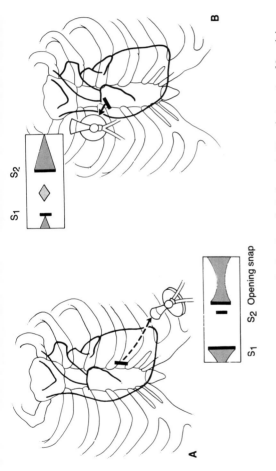

Figure 10–37   Diastolic murmurs. *A*, Pathophysiology of mitral stenosis. Note the intensity of S₁ and the accentuation of the diastolic murmur in late diastole. *B*, Aortic regurgitation. Note the systolic flow murmur. (PMI = point of maximum impulse.)

TABLE 10–23   Resting Average Heart Rates of Infants and Children

Age of Child	Average Heart Rate (beats/min)
Birth	150 ± 50
1–6 months	135 ± 50
7–12 months	115 ± 40
1–2 years	110 ± 40
3–6 years	105 ± 35
7–10 years	95 ± 30
11–15 years	85 ± 30

TABLE 10–24   Differentiation of Breast Masses

Characteristic	Cystic Disease	Benign Adenoma	Malignant Tumor
Patient age	25–60	10–55	25–85
Number	1 or more	1	1
Shape	Round	Round	Irregular
Consistency	Elastic, soft to hard	Firm	Stony hard
Delimitation	Well delimited	Well delimited	Poorly delimited
Mobility	Mobile	Mobile	Fixed
Tenderness	Present	Absent	Absent
Skin retraction	Absent	Absent	Present

TABLE 10–25   Differential Diagnosis of Common Scrotal Swellings

Diagnosis	Usual Age (yr)	Transillumination	Scrotal Erythema	Pain
Epididymitis	Any	No	Yes	Severe
Torsion of testis	20	No	Yes	Severe, sudden
Testis tumor	15–35	No	No	Minimal
Hydrocele (see Fig. 16–23, p. 409)†	Any	Yes (see Fig. 16–24, p. 409)†	No	None
Spermatocele	Any	Yes	No	None
Hernia (see Figs. 16–34, 16–35, p. 415)†	Any	No	No	None to moderate*
Varicocele (see Fig. 16–22, p. 408)†	>15	No	No	No

*Unless incarcerated, at which time pain may be severe.
†In *Textbook of Physical Diagnosis.*

TABLE 10–26   Differential Diagnosis of Genital Papules

Condition	Appearance	Pain	Lymphadenopathy
Herpes	Multiple, ulcers, vesicles	Painful	Present
Condylomata lata (see Fig. 16–33, p. 415)*	Multiple, moist, flat, round	Painful	Present
Condylomata acuminata (see Fig. 16–16, p. 405)*	Multiple, verrucous	Absent	Absent
Molluscum contagiosum (see Figs. 16–30 and 16–31, p. 414)*	1–5 mm umbilicated papules, often in clusters; caseous material expressible from center	Painful	Rarely

*In *Textbook of Physical Diagnosis.*

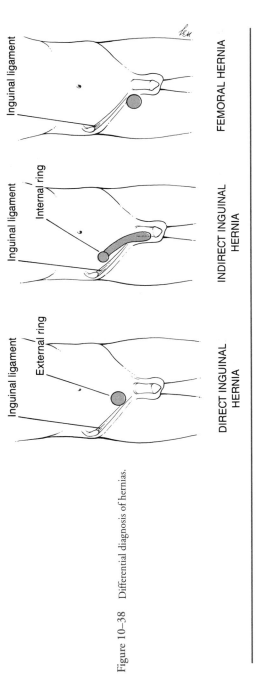

Figure 10–38 Differential diagnosis of hernias.

Feature	Direct Inguinal*	Indirect Inguinal†	Femoral
Occurrence	Middle-aged and elderly men	All ages	Least common; more frequently found in women
Bilaterality	55%	30%	Rarely
Origin of swelling	Above inguinal ligament. Directly behind and through external ring.	Above inguinal ligament. Hernial sac enters inguinal canal at internal ring and exits at external ring.	Below inguinal ligament
Scrotal involvement	Rarely	Commonly	Never
Impulse location	At side of finger in inguinal canal	At tip of finger in inguinal canal	Not felt by finger in inguinal canal; mass below canal

*See Figure 16–35, p. 415, in *Textbook of Physical Diagnosis.*
†See Figure 16–34, p. 415, in *Textbook of Physical Diagnosis.*

TABLE 10–27 Characteristics of Common Vaginal Discharges

Feature	Physiologic Discharge	Nonspecific Vaginitis (NSV)
Color	White	Gray
Fishy odor	Absent	Present
Consistency	Nonhomogeneous	Homogeneous
Present	Dependent	Adherent to walls
Discharge at introitus	Rare	Common
Vulva	Normal	Normal
Vaginal mucosa	Normal	Normal
Cervix	Normal	Normal

TABLE 10–28 Clinical Features of Genital Ulcerations

Feature	Genital Herpes*
Incubation period	3–5 days
Number of ulcers	Multiple
Appearance at onset	Vesicle
Later appearance	Small, grouped
Ulcer pain	Present
Inguinal adenopathy	Present, tender
Healing	Within 2 weeks
Recurrence (even if not infected)	Common

*See Figure 17–28, p. 444, in *Textbook of Physical Diagnosis*.
†See Figure 17–29, p. 444, in *Textbook of Physical Diagnosis*.

Trichomonas	Candida	Gonococcal
Grayish yellow	White	Greenish yellow
Present	Absent	Absent
Purulent, often with bubbles	Cottage cheese–like	Mucopurulent
Often pooled in fornix	Adherent to walls	Adherent to walls
Common	Common	Common
Edematous	Erythematous	Erythematous
Usually normal	Erythematous	Normal
May show red spots	Patches of discharge	Pus in os

Primary Syphilis†		Chancroid
10–90 days		1–5 days
Single		Multiple
Papule		Papule/pustule
Round, indurated		Irregular, ragged
Absent		Present
Present, painless		Present, painful
Slowly over weeks		Slowly over weeks
Rare		Common

TABLE 10–29   Clinical Features Differentiating Rheumatoid Arthritis from Osteoarthritis

Clinical Feature	Rheumatoid Arthritis*	Osteoarthritis†
Patient's age (yr)	3–80	Over 45
Morning stiffness	More than 1 hr	Less than 1 hr
Disability	Often great	Variable
Joint distribution		
Distal interphalangeal joint	Rare	Very common
Proximal interphalangeal joint	Very common	Common
Metacarpophalangeal joint	Very common	Absent
Wrist	Very common	Absent
Soft tissue swelling	Very common	Rare
Interosseous muscle wasting	Very common	Rare
Swan-necking	Common	Rare
Ulnar deviation	Common	Absent

*See Figures 18–55 and 18–56, p. 484, in *Textbook of Physical Diagnosis.*
†See Figure 18–57, p. 485, in *Textbook of Physical Diagnosis.*

TABLE 10–30 Cranial Nerves

Cranial Nerve	Function	Clinical Findings with Lesion
I: Olfactory	Smell	Anosmia
II: Optic	Vision	Amaurosis
III: Oculomotor	Eye movements; pupillary constriction; accommodation	Diplopia; prosis; mydriasis; loss of accommodation
IV: Trochlear	Eye movements	Diplopia
V: Trigeminal	General sensation of face, scalp, and teeth; chewing movements	"Numbness" of face; weakness of jaw muscles
VI: Abducens	Eye movements	Diplopia
VII: Facial	Taste; general sensation of palate and external ear; lacrimal gland, and submandibular and sublingual gland secretion; facial expression	Loss of taste on anterior two thirds of tongue; dry mouth; loss of lacrimation; paralysis of facial muscles
VIII: Vestibulocochlear	Hearing; equilibrium	Deafness; tinnitus; vertigo; nystagmus
IX: Glossopharyngeal	Taste; general sensation of pharynx and ear; elevates palate; parotid gland secretion	Loss of taste on posterior one third of tongue; anesthesia of pharynx; partially dry mouth
X: Vagus	Taste; general sensation of pharynx, larynx, and ear; swallowing; phonation; parasympathetic to heart and abdominal viscera	Dysphagia; hoarseness; palatal paralysis
XI: Spinal accessory	Phonation; head, neck, and shoulder movements	Hoarseness; weakness of head, neck, and shoulder muscles
XII: Hypoglossal	Tongue movements	Weakness and wasting of tongue

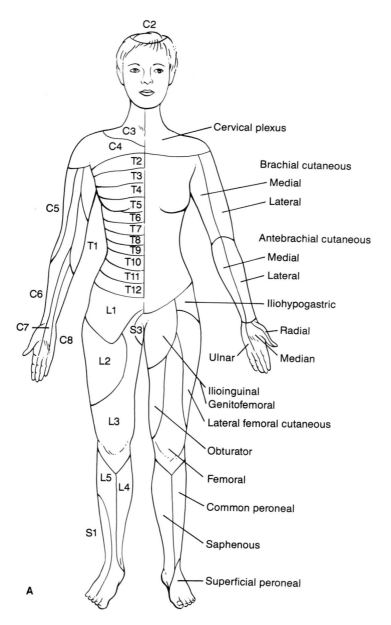

Figure 10–39   Segmental distribution of the spinal nerves. *A*, Distribution in the front.

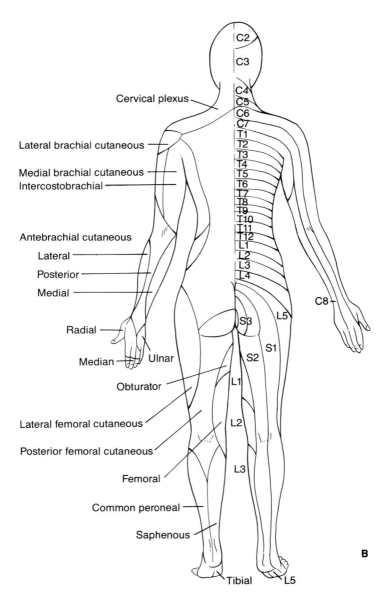

Figure 10–39 **Continued** *B*, Distribution in the back.

TABLE 10–31 Differential Diagnosis of Headache

Type	Epidemiology	Location	Signs and Symptoms
Migraine	Family history Young adults Females	Bifrontal	Nausea Vomiting Possible neurologic deficits
Cluster	Adolescent males	Orbitofrontal Unilateral	Unilateral nasal congestion Lacrimation
Tension	Females	Bilateral Generalized or occipital	
Hypertensive	Family history	Variable	Hypertensive retinopathy Possible papilledema
Increased intracranial pressure		Variable	Nausea Vomiting Papilledema
Meningitis		Bilateral Often occipital	Nuchal rigidity Fever
Temporal arteritis*	Adults	Unilateral Over temporal artery	Tender temporal artery Loss of vision in ipsilateral eye

*See p. 652 in *Textbook of Physical Diagnosis.*

**TABLE 10–32   Common Neurologic Conditions and Their
Signs and Symptoms**

Condition	Age at Onset (yr)	Sex	Signs and Symptoms
Multiple sclerosis	30-35	Women	Nystagmus Diplopia Slurring of speech Muscular weakness Paresthesias Poor coordination Bowel and bladder dysfunction
Amyotrophic lateral sclerosis	50-80	Men	Irregular twitching of involved muscles Muscular weakness Muscle atrophy* Absence of sensory or mental deficits
Parkinson's disease	60-80	Men	Rigidity Slowing of movements Involuntary tremor Difficulty in swallowing Tremor in upper extremities Jerky, "cogwheel" motions Slow, shuffling gait with loss of arm swing Masklike facial expression Body in moderate flexion Excessive salivation
Myasthenia gravis	20-50	Women	Generalized muscular fatigue Bilateral ptosis† Diplopia Difficulty in swallowing Voice weakness
Huntington's chorea	35-50	Both sexes	Choreiform movements Brain failure Rapid movements Facial grimacing Dysarthria Personality change

*See Figure 19–21, p. 521, in *Textbook of Physical Diagnosis.*
†See Figure 8–19, p. 166, in *Textbook of Physical Diagnosis.*

TABLE 10–33   Motor Involvement in Spinal Cord Lesions

Affected Cord Segment	Motor Involvement
C1–4	Paralysis of neck, diaphragm, intercostals, and all four extremities
C5	Spastic paralysis of trunk, arms, and legs; partial shoulder control
C6–7	Spastic paralysis of trunk and legs; upper arm control; partial lower arm control
C8	Spastic paralysis of trunk and legs; hand weakness only
T1–10	Spastic paralysis of trunk and legs
T11–12	Spastic paralysis of legs
L1–S1	Flaccid paralysis of legs
S2–5	Flaccid paralysis of lower legs; bowel, bladder, and sexual function affected

TABLE 10–34   Motor Function According to Cord Segments

Area of Body	Action Tested	Cord Segment
Shoulder	Flexion, extension, or rotation of neck	C1–C4
Arm	Adduction of arm	C5–C8, T1
	Abduction of arm	C4–C6
	Flexion of forearm	C5–C6
	Extension of forearm	C6–C8
	Supination of forearm	C5–C7
	Pronation of forearm	C6–C7
Hand	Extension of hand	C6–C8
	Flexion of hand	C7–C8, T1
Finger	Abduction of thumb	C7–C8, T1
	Adduction of thumb	C8, T1
	Abduction of little finger	C8, T1
	Opposition of thumb	C8, T1
Hip	Flexion of hip	L1–L3
	Extension of leg	L2–L4
	Flexion of leg	L4–L5, S1–S2
	Adduction of thigh	L2–L4
	Abduction of thigh	L4–L5, S1–S2
	Medial rotation of thigh	L4–L5, S1
	Lateral rotation of thigh	L4–L5, S1–S2
	Flexion of thigh	L4–L5
Foot	Dorsiflexion of foot	L4–L5, S1
	Plantar flexion of foot	L5, S1–S2
Toe	Extension of great toe	L4–L5, S1
	Flexion of great toe	L5, S1–S2
	Spreading of toes	S1–S2

TABLE 10–35 Cardiovascular Murmurs of Childhood

Condition	Cycle	Location	Radiation	Pitch	Other Signs
Ventricular septal defect	Pansystolic	Left sternal border at the fourth or fifth intercostal space	Over the precordium, rarely to the axilla	High	Thrill at left lower sternal border
Mitral insufficiency	Pansystolic	Apex	Axilla	High	S_1 decreased S_3
Pulmonic stenosis	Systolic ejection	Left second or third intercostal space	Left shoulder	Medium	Widely split S_2 Right-sided S_4 Ejection click
Patent ductus arteriosus	Continuous	Left second intercostal space	Left clavicle	Medium	Machinery-like, harsh Thrill
Venous hum	Continuous	Medial third of clavicles, often on the right	First and second intercostal spaces	Low	Can be obliterated by pressure on the jugular veins

TABLE 10–36 Exanthematous Diseases of Childhood

Disease	Cutaneous Lesion	Location	Mucous Membranes	Systemic Components
Chickenpox (varicella)	Maculopapular; "tear-drop" vesicles on an erythematous base	Trunk, face, and scalp; centrifugal* spread	Yes	Mild febrile disorder; malaise; rash preceded by a 24 hr prodrome of headache and malaise; all stages and sizes of lesions found at the same time and in the same area; pruritus
Measles (rubeola)	Erythematous, maculopapular, purplish red	Scalp, hairline, forehead, behind ears, upper neck; rash starts on head and spreads rapidly to upper extremities and then to lower extremities; rash often slightly hemorrhagic; as rash fades, brown discoloration occurs and then disappears within 7–10 days	Yes†	Prodrome of 3–4 days of high fever, chills, headache, malaise, cough, photophobia, conjunctivitis; 2 days before the rash develops, Koplik's spots may be seen
Rubella (German measles)	Rose pink, small, irregular macules and papules; rash is the first evidence of the disease	Hairline, face, neck, trunk, extremities; centripetal‡ spread; rapidly involves body in 24 hr and tends to fade as it spreads	Yes	Mild fever present, if any; headache, sore throat, mild upper respiratory infection; presence of suboccipital and posterior auricular lymph nodes

Disease	Description of Rash	Location	Desquamation	Other Signs and Symptoms
Erythema infectiosum (see Fig. 22–29)||	Erythematous malar blush	Face, upper arm, thighs; sudden rash in an asymptomatic child giving a "slapped cheek" appearance; maculopapular rash on upper extremities the next day; several days later, a lacy rash on proximal extremities	No	Mild fever, mild pruritus
Roseola infantum (exanthema subitum)	Macules, rose pink, 2–3 mm; rash appears at end of febrile period; duration of rash only 24 hr	Trunk	Rarely	Sudden onset; high fever
Scarlet fever	Fine, punctate, erythematous lesion that blanches on pressure	Face, along skin folds, buttocks, sternum, between scapulae	Yes	Disease results from toxin produced by group A streptococci as a result of pharyngeal infection¶; abrupt onset of fever, headache, sore throat, vomiting; 12–48 hr later, rash appears

*Moving outward from the center.
†Koplik's spots are highly diagnostic; these appear on the buccal mucosa opposite the first molar teeth; they often appear as blue-white pinpoint papules on an erythematous base.
‡Moving toward the center.
§Forschheimer's sign consists of petechiae or reddish spots on the soft palate during the first day of the illness.
||In *Textbook of Physical Diagnosis.*
¶Bright red lesions, often on tonsils and soft palate.

The Patient's Record

CHAPTER 11

The Clinical Record

It is much more important to know what kind of patient a disease has than
what kind of disease a patient has.
Sir William Osler
1849–1919

The patient's medical record is a legal document. Comments regarding the patient's behavior or attitudes should *not* be part of the record unless they are important from a medical or scientific standpoint. You should describe all parts of the examination that you have performed and indicate those which you have not. A statement such as "The examination of the eye is normal" is much less accurate than "The fundus is normal." In the first case, it is not clear whether the examiner actually attempted to look at the fundus. If a part of the examination is not performed, state that it was "deferred" for whatever reason.

The following describes a complete history and physical examination of a 42-year-old man.

 Patient: John Doe
Date: August 19, 1997

HISTORY

Source

Self, reliable.

Chief Complaint

"Chest pain for the past six months."

History of Present Illness

This is the first Mount Hope admission for this 42-year-old lawyer with atherosclerotic coronary artery disease. The patient's history of chest pain began 4 years before admission. He described the pain as a "dull ache" in the retrosternal area with radiation to his left arm. The pain was provoked by exertion and emotions. On July 15, 1996, Mr. Doe suffered his first heart attack while playing tennis. He had an uneventful hospitalization in King's Hospital in New York City. After 2 weeks in the hospital and 3 weeks at home, he returned to work. The patient suffered a second heart attack 6 months later, again while playing tennis. The patient was hospitalized in King's

Hospital, during which time he was told of an "irregularity" of his heart rate. Since then, the patient has not experienced any palpitations, nor has he been told of any further irregularities.

During the past 6 months, Mr. Doe has noted an increase in the frequency of his chest pain. The pain occurs now four or five times a day and is relieved within 5 minutes with one or two nitroglycerin tablets under his tongue. The pain is produced by exercise, emotions, and sexual intercourse. The patient also describes 1-block dyspnea on exertion. The patient relates that 6 months ago he could walk 2 to 3 blocks before becoming short of breath.

Although the patient shows significant denial of his illness, he is anxious and depressed.

The patient has currently been admitted for elective cardiac catheterization.

Past Medical History
General History

Good.

Past Illnesses

History of untreated hypertension for years (blood pressure not known); no history of measles, chickenpox, mumps, diphtheria, or whooping cough.

Injuries

None.

Hospitalizations

Appendectomy, age 15, Booth Hospital in Rochester, New York (Dr. Meyers, surgeon).

Surgery

See Hospitalizations, above.

Allergies

None.

Immunizations

Salk vaccine for polio, tetanus vaccine, both as a child; no adverse reactions remembered.

Substance Abuse

History of smoking, 40 pack-years (2 packs a day for 20 years); stopped smoking after first heart attack; marijuana on rare occasions in past; drinks alcohol "socially" but also admits to having the need to have a drink as the day goes on (CAGE score, Chapter 1); denies use of other street drugs.

Diet

Mostly red meat, with little fish in diet; 3 cups of coffee a day; recent decrease in appetite, with a 10-pound weight loss in past 3 months.

Sleep Patterns

Recently, falls asleep normally but awakens around 3 AM and cannot go back to sleep.

Current Medications

- Propranolol SR (Inderal), 120 mg daily
- Isosorbide dinitrate (Isordil), 20 mg qid
- Nitroglycerin, 1/150 grains prn
- Chlorpheniramine maleate (Chlor-Trimeton) for colds
- Aspirin for headaches
- Multivitamins with iron daily

Family History (Fig. 11–1)

- Father, 75, diabetes, broken hip
- Mother died, 64, stomach cancer
- Brother, 45, heart attack at age 40
- Sister, 37, alive and well
- Son, 10, alive and well
- Wife, 41, alive and well

There is no family history of congenital disease. No other history of diabetes or cardiac disease. No history of renal, hepatic, or neurologic disease. No history of mental illness.

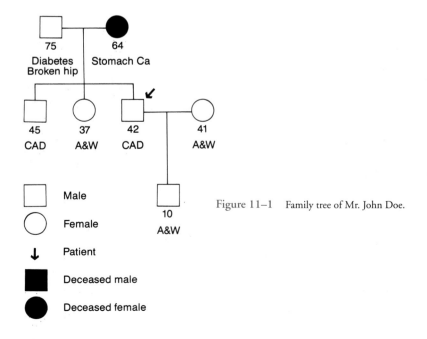

Figure 11–1   Family tree of Mr. John Doe.

Psychosocial History

"Type A" personality; born and raised in Middletown, New York; family moved to Rochester, New York, when Mr. Doe was 13 years old; patient moved to New York City after high school; college and law school in New York City; senior partner of a law firm where he has worked for the past 17 years; married to Emily for the past 13 years; was an active tennis player before second heart attack; before 6 months ago, enjoyed the theater and reading.

Sexual, Reproductive, and Gynecologic History

Patient is male and exclusively heterosexual with one partner, his wife. He has one son, age 10. Recently, because of angina, the patient has stopped having sexual relations.

Review of Systems

General

Depressed for the past 6 months as a result of his ill health.

Skin

No rashes or other changes.

Head

No history of head injury.

Eyes

Wears glasses for reading; no changes in vision recently, saw ophthalmologist 1 year ago for routine examination; no history of eye pain, tearing, discharge, or halos around lights.

Ears

Patient not aware of any problem hearing; no dizziness, discharge, or pain present.

Nose

Occasional cold, two or three times a year, lasting 3 to 5 days; no hay fever or sinus symptoms.

Mouth and Throat

Occasional sore throats and canker sores associated with colds; no difficulty in chewing or eating; brushes and flosses twice a day; sees dentist twice a year; no gingival bleeding.

Neck

No masses or tenderness.

Chest

History of occasional blood-tinged sputum and cough in the morning when patient was smoking, not recently; last chest x-ray study 1 year ago, was told that findings were normal; 1-block dyspnea on exertion (as noted in History of Present Illness, above); no history of wheezing, asthma, bronchitis, or tuberculosis.

Breasts

No masses or nipple discharge noted.

Cardiac

As noted in History of Present Illness, above.

Vascular

No history of cerebrovascular accidents or claudication.

Gastrointestinal

Recent decrease in appetite, with 10-pound weight loss in past few months; uses no laxatives; no history of diarrhea, constipation, nausea, or vomiting; no bleeding noted.

Genitourinary

Urinates four or fives times a day; urine is light yellow, never red; nocturia × 1; no change in stream; no history of urinary infections; no sexual intercourse in past 6 months, owing to angina during sex; no history of venereal disease.

Musculoskeletal

No joint or bone symptoms; no weakness; no history of back problems or gout.

Neurologic

No history of seizures or difficulties in walking or balance; no history of motor or sensory symptoms.

Endocrine

No known thyroid nodules; no history of temperature intolerance; no hair changes; no history of polydipsia or polyuria.

Psychiatric

Depressed and very anxious about his ill health; also anxious about the results of the upcoming cardiac catheterization; asked "What's going to happen to me?"

PHYSICAL EXAMINATION

General Appearance

The patient is a 42-year-old, slightly obese white man, who is lying in bed. He appears slightly older than his stated age. He is in no acute distress but is very nervous. He is well groomed, cooperative, and alert.

Vital Signs

Blood pressure (BP), 175/95/80 right arm (supine), 175/90/85 left arm (supine), 170/90/80 left arm (sitting), 185/95/85 right leg (prone); heart rate, 100 and regular; respirations, 14.

Skin

Pink; no cyanosis present; five to seven nevi (0.5 to1.5 cm in diameter each) on back, most with hair; normal male escutcheon.

Head

Normocephalic, without signs of trauma.

Eyes

Visual acuity with reading glasses using near card: right eye (OD) 20/40, left eye (OS) 20/30; confrontation visual fields full bilaterally; extraocular movements (EOMs) intact; pupils are equal, round, and reactive to light and to accommodation (PERRLA); eyebrows normal; conjunctivae pink; discs sharp; marked arteriovenous (AV) nicking present bilaterally; copper wiring present bilaterally; a cotton-wool spot is present at 1 o'clock position (superior nasal) in the right eye and at 5 o'clock position (inferior temporal) in the left eye; no hemorrhages are present.

Ears

Normal position; no tenderness present; external canals normal; on Rinne test, air conduction > bone conduction (AC > BC) bilaterally; on Weber test, no lateralization; both tympanic membranes appear normal, with normal landmarks clearly seen.

Nose

Straight, without masses; patent bilaterally; mucosa pink, without discharge; inferior turbinates appear normal.

Sinuses

No tenderness present over frontal or maxillary sinuses.

Throat

Lips pink; buccal mucosa pink; all teeth in good condition, without obvious caries; gingivae normal, without bleeding; tongue midline and without masses; uvula elevates in midline; gag reflex intact; posterior pharynx normal.

Neck

Supple, with full range of motion; trachea at midline and freely mobile; no adenopathy present; thyroid not felt; prominent "a" wave seen in neck veins while lying at 45 degrees; neck veins flat while sitting upright.

Chest

Normal anteroposterior (AP) diameter; symmetric excursion bilaterally; normal tactile fremitus bilaterally; chest resonant bilaterally; clear on percussion and auscultation.

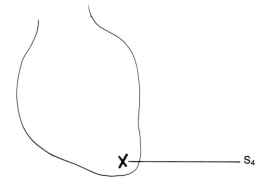

Figure 11–2   Diagram showing location of abnormal cardiac findings.

Breasts

Normal male, without masses, gynecomastia, or discharge.

Heart

Point of maximum impulse (PMI), fifth intercostal space, midclavicular line (5ICS-MCL); S_1 and S_2 normal; normal physiologic splitting present; a loud S_4 is present at the cardiac apex; no murmurs or rubs are heard (Fig. 11–2).

Vascular

Pulses present and symmetric down to the dorsalis pedis bilaterally; no bruits present over the carotid or femoral arteries; no abdominal bruits present; no edema present.

Abdomen

Well-healed appendectomy scar in right lower quadrant (RLQ); abdomen slightly obese; no masses present; no tenderness, guarding, rigidity, or rebound present.

Rectal

Anal sphincter normal; no hemorrhoids present; prostate slightly enlarged and soft; no prostatic masses felt; no stool in ampulla.

Genitalia

Circumcised man with normal genitalia; penis normal and without induration; testicles, 4 × 3 × 2 cm (right) and 3 × 6 × 4 cm (left), with normal consistency.

Lymphatic

No adenopathy noted.

Musculoskeletal

Several stony hard, slightly yellowish, nontender masses over extensor tendons on patient's hands; normal range of motion of neck, spine, and major joints of upper and lower extremities.

TABLE 11–1   Deep Tendon Reflexes of Patient John Doe

	Biceps	Triceps	Knee	Achilles Tendon
Right	2+	2+	2+	1+
Left	2+	2+	1+	1+

Neurologic

Oriented to person, place, and time; cranial nerves II to XII intact (cranial nerve I not tested); cerebellar function normal; plantar reflexes down; gait normal; deep tendon reflexes as in Table 11–1.

SUMMARY

Mr. Doe is a "type A" 42-year-old man with a history of two myocardial infarctions in the past whose current admission is for elective cardiac catheterization. His risk factors for coronary artery disease are untreated hypertension and a long history of cigarette smoking. The patient also has a brother who suffered a myocardial infarction at the age of 40 years.

Physical examination reveals a slightly obese man with hypertension and its associated early to intermediate funduscopic changes. Cardiac examination reveals a loud fourth heart sound, suggestive of a noncompliant (stiff) ventricle. This may be a manifestation of ischemic heart disease or ventricular hypertrophy secondary to the hypertension. Although the patient is not aware of any lipid abnormalities, numerous tendinous xanthomata are present. These are strongly suggestive of hypercholesterolemia, an additional risk factor for premature coronary artery disease.

The problem list containing all the health problems identified, with their dates of recognition and resolution for Mr. Doe, might look like Table 11–2. The problems in

TABLE 11–2   Problem List for Patient John Doe

Problem	Date	Resolved
1. Chest pain	1996	
2. Myocardial infarction	July 15, 1996	2 weeks later
3. Myocardial infarction	January 1997	3 weeks later
4. Hypertension	Years	
5. Smoking	1976	July 15, 1996
6. Tendinous xanthomata	?	
7. S_4 gallop		
8. Dyspnea on exertion	6 months ago	
9. Depression Weight loss Sleeping abnormality	3 months ago	
10. Diet modification		

the list are then used each time the patient is subsequently seen and examined. For each problem, the student or physician should develop a strategy for its ultimate resolution. Each problem should have the following four components:

- **Subjective data**
- **Objective data**
- **Assessment**
- **Plan**

This is the SOAP format,* which contains an update of the subjective and objective data as well as the assessment of the problem and the plan for its resolution.

*Weed LL: Medical records that guide and teach. N Engl J Med 278:593, 652, 1967.

Spanish-Speaking
Patient

CHAPTER 12

English-to-Spanish Translations Useful in the Medical Setting

A physician is obligated to consider more than a diseased organ,
more even than the whole man—he must view the man in his world.

Harvey Cushing
1869–1939

This chapter includes some of the basic words and phrases often needed when one is interviewing and examining a Spanish-speaking person. It includes dialogs using words and expressions for many situations. Most of the questions are written as direct questions and have either *yes* or *no* answers. The phrases and vocabulary presented here will enable the reader to communicate quickly and effectively. **If the pronunciation is too difficult for you, just show the Spanish expression to the patient.**

Spanish is a language that is pronounced approximately as it is written. There are several exceptions:

"c" before "a," "o," "u," or consonant is hard like "c" in *camera*

"c" before "e" or "i" is soft and pronounced like "c" in *receive*

"cc" is pronounced like a "ks" sound like in *accent*

"g" before "a," "o," or "u," is hard like "g" in *great*

"g" before "e" or "i" is breathy like "h" in *home*

"h" is always silent

"j" is breathy and pronounced like "h" in *humid*

"ll" is pronounced like "y" in *yellow*

"ñ" is pronounced like "ny" in *canyon*

"qu" is pronounced like "k" in *key*

"v" is pronounced like "b" in *book*

"z" is pronounced like "s" in *shoe*

Words ending in a vowel "n," or "s" are stressed on the next-to-last syllable. Words ending in a consonant are stressed on the last syllable. A written accent is used on any word that breaks either of these two rules.

A question is preceded by an inverted question mark (¿) at its beginning and a question mark (?) at its end.

BASIC VOCABULARY	VOCABULARIO BASICO
Hello!	¡Hola!
Please	Por favor
Yes	Sí
No	No
Maybe	Quizás
Thank you (very much).	(Muchas) gracias.
You're welcome.	De nada.
Excuse me.	Perdón.
I'm sorry.	Lo siento.
Sir	Señor
Madame	Señora
Miss	Señorita
Please answer either "yes" or "no if you can.	Por favor conteste "sí" o "no" si puede.
What is your name?	¿Cómo se llama usted?
Do you speak English?	¿Habla usted inglés?
Do you understand English?	¿Comprende usted inglés?
Repeat, please.	Repita, por favor.
Please speak more slowly.	Por favor, hable más despacio.
Do you need something?	¿Necesita algo?
Do you want something?	¿Desea algo?
Please speak louder.	Por favor, hable en voz más alta.
What is the name of your doctor?	¿Cuál es el nombre de su médico?
What is his telephone number?	¿Cuál es su número de teléfono?
Good morning.	Buenos días.
Good afternoon.	Buenas tardes.
Good evening.	Buenas noches.
Let me introduce myself.	Déjeme presentarme.
My name is _____.	Me llamo _____.
I am _____.	Soy _____.
What is your name?	¿Cómo se llama usted?
I am glad to meet you.	Me alegro de conocerle.
How are you?	¿Cómo está usted?
How do you feel today?	¿Cómo se siente hoy?
Fair.	Así, así.

May I ask your age?	¿Qué edad tiene usted?
I feel okay.	Me siento bien.
I feel bad.	Me siento mal.
I feel better.	Me siento mejor.
I feel worse.	Me siento peor.
Do you understand?	¿Comprende usted ?
I understand.	Yo comprendo.
I don't understand.	No comprendo.
What? What did you say?	¿Cómo?
When?	¿Cuándo?
Who?	¿Quién?
I don't feel well.	No me siento bien.
Goodbye.	Adiós.
See you later.	Hasta la vista.
I'll see you.	Nos veremos.
See you tomorrow.	Hasta mañana.

What relation is the person to you?

¿Qué parentesco tiene esta persona con usted?

Wife	Esposa
Husband	Esposo
Mother	Madre
Father	Padre
Mother-in-law	Suegra
Father-in-law	Suegro
Son	Hijo
Daughter	Hija
Brother	Hermano
Sister	Hermana
Friend	Amigo
Employer	Patrón

Days of the Week

Días de la Semana

Sunday	El domingo
Monday	El lunes

Tuesday	El martes
Wednesday	El miércoles
Thursday	El jueves
Friday	El viernes
Saturday	El sábado

Seasons of the Year — Las Estaciones

Spring	La primavera
Summer	El verano
Autumn	El otoño
Winter	El invierno

Months of the Year — Los Meses del Año

January	Enero
February	Febrero
March	Marzo
April	Abril
May	Mayo
June	Junio
July	Julio
August	Agosto
September	Septiembre
October	Octubre
November	Noviembre
December	Diciembre

Expressions of Time — Expressions de Horario

Today	Hoy
Yesterday	Ayer
Tomorrow	Mañana
Tonight	Esta noche
Now	Ahora
The day after tomorrow	Pasado mañana
The day before yesterday	Anteayer
A week from today	En una semana de hoy
Every other day	Cada otro día
Month	Mes

Week	Semana
Year	Año
Next week	La semana que viene
Next month	El mes que viene
Next year	El año que viene
Minute	Minuto
Daily	Diario
Weekly	Semanal
Monthly	Mensual (mensualmente)
Yearly	Anual (anualmente)
Year round	Todo el año
During the day	Durante el día
First time	Primera vez
Last time	Última vez
Once	Una vez
Once a day	Una vez al día
Twice a day	Dos veces al día
Three times a day	Tres veces al día
Four times a day	Cuatro veces al día
How often?	¿Con qué frecuencia?
How many times?	¿Cúantas veces?
Early	Temprano
Late	Tarde
Every hour	A cada hora
Every two hours	Cada dos horas
Constantly	Constantemente
Sometimes	A veces
Often	A menudo
On time	A tiempo
Per day	Al (por) día
Per month	Al (por) mes
Per week	A (por) la semana
At bedtime	Al acostarse
Upon getting up	Al levantarse
At the same time	A la misma vez
From time to time	De vez en cuando
Immediately	Inmediatamente

Lately	Últimamente
Moment	Momento
Second	Segundo
Before meals	Antes de comer
After meals	Después de comer
In a few minutes	Dentro de poco minutos
Since when?	¿Desde cúando?
For how long?	¿Por cúanto tiempo
For many years	Por muchos años
For the time being	Por ahora

Patient Complaints / Problemas del Paciente

abscess	un absceso
broken bone	un hueso roto
bruise	una contusión
burn	una quemadura
chills	escalofrío
cold	un catarro
constipation	estreñimiento
stomach cramps	calambres
diarrhea	diarrea
fever	fiebre
headache	dolor de cabeza
infection	infección
lump	un bulto
sore throat	dolor de garganta
stomach ache	dolor de estómago

Parts of the Body / Partes del Cuerpo

ankle	el tobillo
appendix	el apéndice
arm	el brazo
back	la espalda
breast	el pecho
cheek	la mejilla

ear	el oído
elbow	el codo
eye	el ojo
face	la cara
finger	el dedo
foot	el pie
glands	las glándulas
hand	la mano
head	la cabeza
heart	el corazón
hip	la cadera
knee	la rodilla
leg	la pierna
lip	el labio
liver	el hígado
mouth	la boca
neck	el cuello
nose	la nariz
shoulder	el hombro
skin	la piel
thumb	el pulgar
throat	la garganta
toe	el dedo del pie
tooth	el diente
wrist	la muñeca

Present Illness

Enfermedad Actual

What problem has brought you to the hospital?

¿Cual problema le ha traido usted a este hospital?

When did you last feel perfectly well?

¿Cúando fue la última vez en que usted se sentio perfectamente bien?

What bothers you the most?

¿Qué le molesta más?

How long have you been ill?

¿Cúanto tiempo hace que usted está enfermo?

an hour
a day
a week

una hora
un día
una semana

a month

a year

Have you had ____? When?
   fever
   cough
   bleeding
   pain

Are you in pain?

When did the pain begin?

Where is the pain?

Show me where it hurts you.

Point to where it hurts.
   In the head?
   In the chest?
   On the side?
   In the back?

Is it a constant pain or does it come and go?

Is your pain (cough, bleeding)
   constant?
   severe?

Is your pain ____?
   cramping?
   stabbing?
   burning?
   aching?

Does the pain occur during ____
   sleep?
   breathing?
   urination?
   bowel movements?
   exertion?

Has the pain changed its location?
   From where to where?

Does the pain radiate? Where to?

Have you taken any drugs? Any medications? What were they?

Did this medicine give you relief?

Had you been in good health before this illness?

un mes

un año

¿Ha tenido usted ____? ¿Cuándo?
   fiebre
   tos
   hemorragia
   dolor

¿Siente usted dolor?

¿Cuándo empezaron sus dolores?

¿Dónde siente dolor?

Enséñeme donde le duele.

Indíqueme dónde le duele.
   ¿En la cabeza?
   ¿En el pecho?
   ¿En un costado?
   ¿En la espalda?

¿Es un dolor constante, o viene y se le va?

¿Es su dolor (tos, hemorragia)…
   constante?
   severa?

¿Es su dolor como ____?
   un calambre?
   una puñalada?
   quemadura?
   simplemente dolor?

¿Aparece el dolor ____
   durante el sueño?
   durante la respiración?
   cuando orina?
   durante la defecación?
   cuando efectúa un esfuerzo?

¿Ha cambiado de sitio el dolor?
   ¿De donde a donde?

¿Se corre el dolor por el cuerpo? A donde?

¿Ha tomado usted drogas? Remedios? Cuáles fueron?

¿Obtuvo usted alivio con esta medicina?

¿Ha gozado usted de buena salud antes de esta enfermedad?

Have you ever been treated in this hospital? When?	¿Ha sido usted tratado en esta hospital? Cuándo?
Have you ever been admitted to any other hospital? When?	¿Ha sido usted admitido en otros hospitales? Cuándo?
Have you ever had any operations? Serious injuries? Please show me.	¿Ha sido usted operado? Heridas de importancia? Por favor enséñeme donde.
Have you ever had any other diseases? What were they?	¿Ha tenido usted otras enfermedades? Cuáles fueron?
Did you have this _____	¿Cuánto tiempo hace que usted ha padecido de estas enfermedades?
days ago	días atrás
weeks ago	semanas atrás
months ago	meses atrás
years ago	años atrás
If anything makes you feel better, show me what it is.	Si algo le mejora, enséñame en que consiste.
Have your symptoms been bad enough to keep you in bed?	¿Eran sus síntomas bastante severos para obligarse a quedarse en cama?
Have you been getting better? Worse?	¿Va usted mejorando? Enpeorando?
Were you in an accident? Show me your injury.	¿Ha sufrido un accidente? Enséñeme donde está herido.
What is the name of your employer?	¿Para qué compañía trabaja usted?
What is the address of your employer?	¿Cuál es la dirección de su trabajo? Donde está usted empleado (empleada)?

Past Medical History

Please answer *yes* or *no* to the following questions:

Have you had any surgery?

When?
Where?
What type?

Have you ever had _____
rheumatic fever?
asthma?

Previa Historia Médica

Por favor de contestar *si* o *no* a las preguntas siguientes:

¿Ha tenido usted algún cirugía (operación)?
¿Cuándo?
¿Dónde?
¿Qué tipo?

¿Ha padecido usted alguna ves de _____
fiebre reumático?
asma?

tuberculosis?

hepatitis?

liver disease?

kidney disease?

heart disease?

lung disease?

stroke?

heart attack?

ulcer?

diabetes?

cancer?

high blood pressure?

allergies?

anemia?

jaundice?

any previous surgery?

Do you take _____

vitamins?

painkillers?

laxatives?

antacids?

expectorants?

antibiotics?

narcotics?

sedatives?

anticonvulsants?

tranquilizers?

anticoagulants?

blood pressure medications?

heart pills?

water pills?

Do you have any allergies?

What medicines are you allergic to?

None

Penicillin

Sulfa

Tetanus

Codeine

Aspirin

tuberculosis?

hepatitis?

enfermedad del higado?

enfermedad del riñon?

enfermedad del corazón?

enfermedad del pulmón?

derrame cerebral?

ataque de corazón?

úlcera?

diabetes?

cancer?

alta presión?

alergia?

anemia?

ictericia (piel amarilla)?

cualquier cirugiá anterior?

¿Usa usted _____

vitaminas?

pildoras par el dolor?

laxativos?

antiácidos?

expectorantes?

antibióticos?

narcóticos

calmantes?

anticonvulsivos?

tranquilizantes?

anticoagulantes?

medicinas para alta presión?

pildoras para el corazón?

pildoras para orinar?

¿Tiene usted alergias?

¿A qué medicinas es usted alérgico?

Ninguna

Penicilina

Sulfa

Tétano

Codeína

Aspirina

Hazardous Exposures

Have you been exposed to _____
    industrial dusts?
    gases?
    vapors?
    chemicals?
    radiation?
    extreme noise?
    extreme vibration?

What type of work do you do?

Does anyone in your family work
    in a trade where hazardous
    materials could have been
    brought home?
    asbestos?
    lead?
    vinyl chloride?

Did you ever live near a(n) _____
    industrial plant?
    shipyard?
    mine?
    other facility that may have
        released hazardous
        material?

Expuestaciones Peligrosas

¿Ha estado expuesta a _____
    polvos industrial?
    gases?
    vapores?
    químicos?
    radiación?
    ruido extremo?
    vibración extrema?

¿Qué clase de trabajo hace usted?

¿Trabaja alguien en su familia en
    algo donde es posible que puedan
    traer material peligroso a la casa?

    ¿asbesto?
    ¿plomo?
    ¿cloruro vinyl?

¿Ha vivido usted cerca de una _____
    planta industrial?
    astillero?
    mina?
    otras facilidades que han
        podido soltar materiales
        peligrosos?

Social History

Where were you born?

Are you married?

Do you smoke?

How much?

For how long?

How often do you drink?
    Beer?
    Wine?
    Hard liquor?

How long has this been your pattern?

Historia Social

¿Dónde nació?

¿Es usted casado (M)? casada (F)?

¿Fuma usted?

¿Cúanto?

¿Por cuánto tiempo?

¿Cúanto bebe?
    ¿Cerveza?
    ¿Vino?
    ¿Bebida alcohólica?

¿Por cuánto tiempo has sido esta
    su costumbre?

Do you use any drugs to make you feel better or change your mood?

¿Usa usted drogas para sentirse mejor o para cambiar su humor?

What?

¿Qué?

How much?

¿Cuánto?

Has your use of drugs or alcohol ever caused you to have problems with _____
family?
health?
job?
finances?

¿Ha presentado su costumbre con el uso de drogas o alcohol problema con _____
familia?
salud?
trabajo?
financiero?

Have you had any problems with the law because of your use of drugs or alcohol?

¿Ha tenido usted algún problema con la ley sobre su uso de drogas/alcohol?

Have you ever sought help for _____

your pattern of drinking?
your use of drugs?

¿Ha tratado usted de conseguir ayuda por _____
su hábito de la bebida?
su uso de drogas?

Have you ever been sexually or physically abused?

¿Ha sido usted abusado alguna vez sexualmente o fisicamente?

Family History

Historia Familial

Is there any family history of _____

diabetes?
high blood pressure?
angina?
heart disease?
lung disease?
cancer?
strokes?
anemia?
nervous problems?
muscular problems?
endocrine problems?
emotional disturbances?

¿Hay alguna historia en su familia de _____

diabetes?
alta presión?
angina?
enfermedad del corazón?
enfermedad de los pulmones?
cancer?
hemorragia vascular?
anemia?
problemas nervioso?
problemas musculares?
problemas de glándulas endocrinas?
disturbios emocionales?

Have you ever been pregnant?

¿Ha estado embarazada?

Do you have any children?

¿Tiene hijos?

How is your health?

¿Cómo está la salud?

Review of Systems

Have you ever had:

General Status

Insomnia
Recent weight loss
Fatigue or weakness
Fever or chills
Sweating, night sweats
Irritability

Skin

Rashes or eruptions
Itching
Hair or nail changes
Easy bruising
Bleeding
Head
Headache
Trauma
Change in hat size
Fainting
Dizziness
Migraine

Eyes

Loss of vision or blurring
Double vision
Do you wear glasses?
Color blindness
Pain or discharge
Redness
Blind spots
Eye pain when looking at lights
Excessive tearing

Revisión de Sistemas

¿Ha padecido alguna vez de:

Estado General

Insomnia
Reciente cambio de peso
Fatiga o debilidad
Fiebre o escalofríos
Sudor, sudor de noche
Irritabilidad

Piel

Ronchas o erupciónes
Picazón
Cambio de cabello o uñas
Golpes leves
Sangrado
Cabeza
Dolor de cabeza
Traumatismo
Cambio de medida de sombrero
Desmayo
Vértigo
Jaqueca

Ojos

Borrón o pérdida de visión
Doble visión
¿Usa usted anteojos?
Daltonismo
Dolor o descargo
Enrojecimiento
Puntos ciegos
Dolor en los ojos cuándo mira a la luz
Lagrimeo excesivo

Ears

Discharge or pain

Deafness (hearing loss)

Vertigo

Ringing in ears

Los Oídos

Le supuran o duelen los oídos

Ensordecimiento (pérdida de audición)

Vértigo

Sonar el oído

Nose

Discharge

Hay fever

Nasal obstruction

Postnasal drip

Nose bleed

Nariz

Supuración

Fiebre del heno

Obstrucción nasal

Goteo posterior nariz

Le sangra la nariz

Mouth, Throat, and Larynx

Sores (ulcers)

How are your teeth?

Dental care

Dentures

Gum bleeding

Taste

Persistent hoarseness

Sore throat

Boca, Garganta y Laringe

Llaga (úlcera)

¿Cómo están sus dientes?

Cuidado dental

Dentadura

Le sangran las encías

Sabor

Ronquera persistente

Dolor de garganta

Pulmonary

Shortness of breath

Wheezing

Stridor

Cough

Sputum

Cough up blood

Pulmonar

Le falta la respiración

Le silba el pecho

Estridor

Tos

Esputo

Tose sangre

Breasts

Masses

Pain

Discharge from nipples

Swelling

Los Pechos (Senos)

Masas

Dolor

Le supuran los pezones

Hinchazón

Have you had bleeding or discharge from the nipples?

¿Le han supurado o sangrado los pezones?

Have you noticed any abnormal change in the breasts?

¿Ha notado algún cambio anormal en los senos?

Cardiovascular

Cardiovascular

Palpitation	Palpitación
Shortness of breath	Falta de respiración
Do you sleep on any pillows?	¿Duerme usted con almohada?
Have you ever awakened in the middle of the night short of breath?	¿Se despierta usted por la noche por falta de respiración?
Chest pain	Dolor de pecho
Cyanosis	Cianosis
History of murmur	Historia de ruido
Hypertension	Alta presión
Edema	Edema
Convulsions	Convulsiones
How many level blocks can you walk before becoming short of breath?	¿Cuántas cuadras puede usted andar antes de sentir falta de respiración?

Gastrointestinal

Gastrointestinal

Change in appetite	Cambio de apetito
Abdominal pain	Dolor abdominal
Difficulty in swallowing	Dificultad tragando
Indigestion	Indigestión
History of jaundice	Historia of ictericia
Hepatitis	Hepatitis
Constipation	Estreñimiento
Diarrhea	Diarrea
Change in bowel habits	Cambio de sus evacuaciones
Change in stool shape and color	Forma y color de evacuaciones
Anal discomfort	Malestar anal
Hemorrhoids	Hemorroides
Nausea	Náusea
Vomiting	Vómito
Hernia	Hernia
Change in abdominal girth	Cambio de medida abdominal
Vomiting of blood	Vómito de sangre

Black, tarry stools	Evacuaciones negras o color de marrón
Belching	Eructación
Bloating	Aventado
Parasites	Parásitos

Genitourinary | ## Genitourinario

Pain on urination	Ardor o dolor cuando urina
Change in urine color	Cambio de color de la urina
Do you awaken from sleep to urinate?	¿Se despierta usted por la noche para orinar?
Have you ever had red urine?	¿Ha tenido usted orina roja?
Do you have any problems starting or stopping urination?	¿Tiene usted problemas comenzando o terminando de orina?
Have you ever had kidney stones?	¿Ha tenido alguna vez cálculos en los riñones?
Have you ever had a kidney infection?	¿Ha tenido alguna vez infección en los riñones?

Sexual History | ## Historia Sexual

Venereal disease	Venéreo enfermedade
Syphilis	Sífilis
Gonorrhea	Gonorrea
Sores	Llagas
Discharge	Supuración
Testicular pain	Dolor testicular
Scrotal swelling	Hinchazón escrotal
Sterility	Esterilidad
Impotence	Impotencia
Methods of contraception	Método de contraceptivo
History of HIV infection?	¿Historia de infección de SIDA?
Are you sexually active?	¿Está activo sexualmente?
Male/female?	¿Hombre/mujer?
Are you having any sexual problems?	¿Tiene usted problema sexual?

Gynecologic | ## Gynecologia

| When was your last period? | ¿Cuándo fue su última menstruación? |
| Age at onset of menstruation | A qué edad usted comenzó su menstruación |

How long does your period last?	¿Cuánto tiempo le dura su menstruación?
How often do you get your period?	¿Cada cuánto tiempo tiene su menstruación?
Please write down the number.	Por favor anote el número.
Spotting	Manchas
Irregularity	Irregularidad
Pain with period	Menstruación con dolor
Hot flashes	Calor/frio
Sweating	Sudor
Vaginal discharge	Secreción vaginal
Vaginal itch	Picor vaginal
Do you use birth control? What do you use?	¿Practica usted el control de la natalidad? ¿Qué usa usted?
Pills	Las pastillas
IUD	Artefacto intrauterino
Diaphragm	Diafragma
Other	Otro
Are your menstrual periods regular?	¿Es usted regular en sus períodos?
Do you think you may be pregnant now?	¿Cree usted que está en estado, o encinta, ahora?
Have you ever had an abortion?	¿Ha tenido algún aborto?

Endocrine

Glándulas Endocrinas

Goiter	Bocio
Tremor	Temblor
Hot/cold intolerance	Intolerancia calor/frio
Diabetes mellitus	Diabetes mellitus
Hormone therapy	Terapia hormonal
Acne	Acne
Change in skin color	Cambio en color de piel

Allergic History

Historia de Alergia

Sensitivity to allergens, drugs, vaccines, foods	Sensitividad o alergias a drogas, vacunas, comidas
Eczema	Eczema
Hives	Ronchas
Asthma	Asma
Hay fever	Fiebre del heno

Neurologic

Unconsciousness

Fainting

Convulsions

Epilepsy

Loss of, or change in, sensation

Gait and coordination

Speech

Paralysis or weakness

Loss of control of urination or defecation

Problems with ejaculation

Problems with erection

Neurologica

Inconsciente (pérdido del sentido)

Desmayo

Convulsiones

Epilepsia

Pérdido de, o cambio en sensación

Paso y coordinación

Palabra

Parálisis o debilidad

Pérdida del control de la orina o defecación

Problemas con eyaculación

Problemas con erección

Psychologic

Memory loss

Mood

Sleep pattern

Anxiety

Depression

Psicológico

Pérdida de memoria

Humor

Manera de dormir

Ansiedad

Depresión

Musculoskeletal

Trauma

Swelling

Arthritis

Leg pain

Back pain

Musculoesqueleto

Traumatismo

Hinchazón

Artritis

Dolor de piernas

Dolor de espalda

Blood, Lymphatic

Anemia

Transfusions

Bleeding tendency

Lymph node enlargement

Sangre, Linfático

Anemia

Transfusiones

Tendencia a sangrar

Aumento de ganglios linfáticos

Physical Examination

You are now going to have a
  physical examination.

Please remove your clothing.

Can you _____ this?
  smell
  taste
  see
  feel
  hear

Without moving your head, follow my
  finger with your eyes.

Look at this spot and try to keep
  your eyes steady.

Turn your head to the right; to the left.

Read these letters for me, please.

Look up.

Look down.

Look at me.

Keep looking at my nose.

Do you hear this tuning fork vibrating?

Do you feel any vibrations now?

Which side do you hear best?

Open your mouth, please.

Stick out your tongue.

Swallow, please.

Turn your head, please.

Take a deep breath. Cough.
  Cough again.

Breathe through your _____
  mouth
  nose

Breathe deeply, please.

Breathe through your mouth,
  slowly.

Examen Físico

Ahora voy a efectuar su examen físico.

Por favor, quítese la ropa.

¿Puede usted _____ esto?
  oler
  gustar (sentir el gusto)
  ver
  sentir
  oir

Sin mover la cabeza, siga mi dedo
  con sus ojos.

Mire este punto trate de mantener
  los ojos firmes.

Mueva la cabeza a la derecha; a la
  izquierda.

Léame estas letras, por favor.

Mire para arriba.

Mire para abajo.

Hacia mí.

Míreme la nariz.

¿Oye este diapasón vibrar?\

¿Siente algunas vibraciones ahora?

¿En que lado oye esto mas claramente?

Abra su boca, por favor.

Saque la lengua.

Traque, por favor.

Mueva la cabeza, por favor.

Respire profundo. Tosa. Tosa
  otra vez.

Respire por su _____
  boca
  nariz

Respire fuerte, por favor.

Respire por la boca, despacio.

Cough, please.	Tosa , por favor.
Please try to relax.	Por favor, tranquilícese.
Relax your muscles.	Relaje sus músculos.
Does it hurt more when I press or when I stop pressing suddenly?	¿Le duele más cuándo le comprimo o cuándo dejo de comprimir?
Does it hurt only where I am pressing or somewhere else?	¿Le duele solamente donde aprieto o en otras lugares más?
I will not hurt you.	No voy a hacerle daño.
Tell me when you feel pain.	Avíseme cuándo sienta dolor.
Stand up.	Levántese.
Sit down.	Siéntese.
Sit up.	Incorporese.
Lie down.	Acuéstese.
Roll over.	Voltearse.
Say "ah."	Diga "ah."
Bend over.	Inclínese.
I have to examine you internally.	Tengo que examinarle por dentro.
I am going to do a pelvic examination.	Voy a hacerle ahora un examen de la pelvis.
Put your feet in these stirrups.	Ponga los pies en estos estribos.
I am going to examine your rectum.	Voy a examinarle el recto.
This is a rectal examination. It's a little uncomfortable.	Le vamos a examinar el recto. Será un poco incómodo.
Please give me a specimen of your _____ urine stool	Haga el favor de darnos una muestra de _____ la orina las heces fecales
Please get dressed.	Por favor, vístase.
Thank you for your time.	Gracias por su tiempo.
Nice to have met you.	Ha sido un verdadero gusto.

Appendix

Acceptable Medical Abbreviations and Symbols

The following is a list of acceptable abbreviations. The list has been carefully selected from the many abbreviations used nationally. Abbreviations should be considered as a convenience and time-saver. Hopefully, they will also serve as a means of avoiding misspelling words. It is most important to recognize, however, that abbreviations are often misinterpreted or misunderstood; they can be dangerous. For example, the abbreviation *AA* may mean acute asthma, Alcoholics Anonymous, alcohol abuse, alveolar-arterial gradient, antiarrhythmic agent, aortic aneurysm, aplastic anemia, or ascending aorta, among others! While *AP* may mean an appendicitis to a surgeon, *AP* may be understood as angina pectoris, atrial pacing, or arterial pressure to the cardiologist, anterior-posterior to the radiologist, antepartum to the gynecologist-obstetrician, or alkaline phosphatase. *MS* is mental status or multiple sclerosis to the neurologist, mitral stenosis or mitral sound to the cardiologist, muscle strength or musculoskeletal to the rheumatologist, neurologist, or orthopedist, or even morphine sulphate! Although *PND* usually means paroxysmal nocturnal dyspnea, physicians in some regional areas recognize this abbreviation as postnasal drip, pelvic node dissection, or pregnancy not delivered! Be careful when using abbreviations. The list that follows indicates abbreviations and their meaning(s).

A

A$_2$ aortic second sound

AAL anterior axillary line

AAO $\times$ **3** awake and oriented to person, place, and time

A > B air conduction greater than bone conduction

AC > BC air conduction greater than bone conduction

ACE angiotensin-converting enzyme

ACTH adrenocorticotropic hormone

ADH antidiuretic hormone

ADL activities of daily living

AF acid-fast
afebrile
anterior fontanel
aortofemoral
atrial fibrillation

AFB acid-fast bacilli
aortofemoral bypass

A fib atrial fibrillation

AFl atrial flutter

AGA acute gonococcal arthritis
appropriate for gestational age

AIDS acquired immunodeficiency syndrome

ALAD abnormal left axis deviation

ALFT abnormal liver function tests

ALK-P alkaline phosphatase

ALL acute lymphoblastic leukemia

ALT alanine transaminase (SGPT)

AMI acute myocardial infarction

AML acute myelogenous leukemia

AMML acute myelomonocytic leukemia

ANA antinuclear antibody

ANG angiogram

ANISO anisocytosis

A & O $\times$ **3** awake and oriented to person, place, and time

A & P active and present
anterior and posterior
assessment and plans
auscultation and percussion

A$_2$ > P$_2$ second aortic sound greater than second pulmonic sound

ARC AIDS-related complex
American Red Cross
ARD acute respiratory disease
acute respiratory distress
aphakic retinal detachment
ARDS adult respiratory distress syndrome
ASA aspirin
ASAP as soon as possible
ASCVD atherosclerotic cardiovascular disease
ASD atrial septal defect
ASD I atrial septal defect, type I (primum)
ASD II atrial septal defect, type II (secundum)
ASH asymmetric septal hypertrophy
ASHD atherosclerotic heart disease
ASMA anti-smooth muscle antibody
ASMI anteroseptal myocardial infarction
AST aspartate transaminase (SGOT)
ATN acute tubular necrosis
AT/NC atraumatic, normocephalic
AUR acute urinary retention
AVB atrioventricular block
AVF arteriovenous fistula
AVH acute viral hepatitis
AVR aortic valve replacement
A & W alive and well
AWMI anterior wall myocardial infarction
AWO airway obstruction

B

Ba barium
B > A bone conduction greater than air conduction
B & A brisk and active
Bab Babinski
BaE barium enema
BAND band neutrophil (stab)
BANS back, arm, neck, and scalp
BASO STIP basophilic stippling
BAVP balloon aortic valvuloplasty
BBB blood brain barrier
bundle branch block
BC birth control
blood culture
Blue Cross
bone conduction
BCG bacille Calmette-Guérin vaccine (tuberculosis)
BCP birth control pills

BDR background retinal retinopathy
BE bacterial endocarditis
barium enema
below elbow
base excess
B & E brisk and equal
BF breast-feed
BG blood glucose
bone graft
BID twice daily
Bili bilirubin
BILI-C conjugated bilirubin
BKA below knee amputation
BLL bilateral lower lobe
BM bone marrow
bowel movement
breast milk
BN bladder neck
BNO bladder neck obstruction
BOE bilateral otitis externa
BOM bilateral otitis media
BOMA bilateral otitis media, acute
BOO bladder outlet obstruction
BOT base of tongue
BP bathroom privileges
bed pan
bipolar
birthplace
blood pressure
bullous pemphigoid
bypass
BPH benign prostatic hypertrophy
BPO bilateral partial oophorectomy
BPR blood per rectum
BPS bilateral partial salpingectomy
BRADY bradycardia
BRAO branch retinal artery occlusion
BRB blood-retinal barrier
BRBR bright red blood per rectum
BRBPR bright red blood per rectum
BRAO branch retinal arterial occlusion
BRVO branch retinal vein occlusion
BSA body surface area
BSO bilateral salpingo-oophorectomy
BSOM bilateral serous otitis media
BSPA bowel sounds present and active
BTL bilateral tubal ligation
BTO bilateral tubal occlusion
BUN blood urea nitrogen
BVL bilateral vas ligation

C

CABG coronary artery bypass graft
CABS coronary artery bypass surgery
CAGE questionnaire for alcoholism evaluation (JAMA 252:1905, 1984)
CAH chronic active hepatitis
Ca/P calcium to phosphate ratio
CAPD chronic ambulatory peritoneal dialysis
CATH catheterization
CCE clubbing, cyanosis, and edema
CCU coronary care unit
critical care unit
CD4 helper-inducer T-cell
CD8 suppressor-cytotoxic T-cell
CEA carcinoembryonic antigen
carotid endarterectomy
CFNS chills, fever, and night sweats
CHL conductive hearing loss
CHB complete heart block
CHF congestive heart failure
CK creatine kinase
CK-BB creatine kinase, BB band
CK-MB creatine kinase, MB band
CK-MM creatine kinase, MM band
CMJ carpometacarpel joint
CML chronic myelogenous leukemia
C/O complained of
COLD chronic obstructive lung disease
COPD chronic obstructive pulmonary disease
CPAP continuous positive airway pressure
CPD cephalopelvic disproportion
chronic peritoneal dialysis
CPH chronic persistent hepatitis
CPK creatinine phosphokinase
CPPV continuous positive pressure ventilation
CPR cardiopulmonary resuscitation
CRAO central retinal artery occlusion
CRBBB complete right bundle branch block
CREST calcinosis, Raynaud's disease, esophageal dysmotility, sclerodactyly, and telangiectasia
CRST calcification, Raynaud's phenomenon, scleroderma, and telangiectasia
CRV central retinal vein
CRVO central retinal vein occlusion
C/S cesarean section
culture and sensitivity
CSCR central serous chorioretinopathy

CTA clear to auscultation
CTAP clear to auscultation and percussion
CVAT costovertebral angle tenderness
CVO central vein occlusion
CVP central venous pressure
C/W consistent with
CXR chest x-ray

D

D&C dilation and curettage
DDx differential diagnosis
DIFF differential blood count
DKA diabetic ketoacidosis
DOA dead on arrival
DOE dyspnea on exertion
DRG diagnosis-related groups
DSA digital subtraction angiography
DTR deep tendon reflexes
DUB dysfunctional uterine bleeding
DVT deep vein thrombosis
Dx diagnosis

E

EBV Epstein-Barr virus
ECD endocardial cushion defect
ECG electrocardiogram
ECHO echocardiogram
ECT electroconvulsive therapy
EDV end-diastolic volume
EEG electroencephalogram
EENT eyes, ears, nose, and throat
EF ejection fraction
erythroblastosis fetalis
EKG electrocardiogram
EMG electromyogram
ER emergency room
ERCP endoscopic retrograde cholangiopancreatography
ERG electroretinogram
ESR erythrocyte sedimentation rate
ESRD end-stage renal disease
ETOH alcohol
ETP elective termination of pregnancy
EUA examination under anesthesia
EUP extrauterine pregnancy

F

FANA fluorescent antinuclear antibody
FBS fasting blood sugar
FCBD fibrocystic breast disease

FEV$_1$ forced expiratory volume in one second
FFB flexible fiberoptic bronchoscopy
FFP fresh frozen plasma
FHR fetal heart rate
FROM full range of motion
FTA fluorescent treponemal antibody
F/U follow-up

G

GBP gated blood pool
GH growth hormone
Grav. gravid (pregnancy)

H

HAA hepatitis-associated antigen
HBV hepatitis B virus
HCC hepatocellular carcinoma
HCG human chorionic gonadotropin
HDL high-density lipoprotein
HEENT head, eyes, ears, nose, and throat
Hgb hemoglobin
HGH human growth hormone
HIV human immunodeficiency virus
HLA human lymphocyte antigen
HOCM hypertrophic obstructive cardiomyopathy
H & P history and physical
HPI history of present illness
HSV herpes simplex virus
HTLV III human T-cell lymphotrophic virus, type III
HTN hypertension
Hx history

I

IABP intra-aortic balloon pump
IACP intra-aortic counterpulsation
IAN intern's admission note
IBD inflammatory bowel disease
ICP intracranial pressure
ICPP intubated continuous positive pressure
ICU intensive care unit
I & D incision and drainage
IDDM insulin-dependent diabetes mellitus
IDDS implantable drug delivery system
IgA immunoglobulin A
IgD immunoglobulin D
IgE immunoglobulin E
IgG immunoglobulin G
IgM immunoglobulin M

IGR intrauterine growth retardation
IHSS idiopathic hypertrophic subaortic stenosis
ILBBB incomplete left bundle branch block
ILMI inferolateral myocardial infarction
IMB intermenstrual bleeding
IMI inferior myocardial infarction
INH isoniazid
I & O intake and output
IOF intraocular fluid
IOL intraocular lens
IOLI intraocular lens implantation
ION ischemic optic neuropathy
IPPB intermittent positive pressure breathing
IPPV intermittent positive pressure ventilation
IRBBB incomplete right bundle branch block
IRDS idiopathic respiratory distress syndrome
ITP idiopathic thrombocytopenic purpura
IUCD intrauterine contraceptive device
IUGR intrauterine growth retardation
IUP intrauterine pregnancy
IUTD immunizations up to date
IV intravenous
IVCD intraventricular conduction defect
IVDA intravenous drug abuse
IVDSA intravenous digital subtraction angiography
IVDU intravenous drug user
IVF *in vitro* fertilization
IVP intravenous pyelogram
IVS intraventricular septum
IVSD intraventricular septal defect
IWMI inferior wall myocardial infarction

J

JODM juvenile onset diabetes mellitus
JR junctional rhythm
JRA juvenile rheumatoid arthritis

K

KS Kaposi's sarcoma
KUB kidney, ureter, and bladder
KVO keep vein open

L

LAD left anterior descending
left axis deviation

LADA left anterior descending artery
LAE left atrial enlargement
LAFB left anterior fascicular block
LAG lymphangiogram
LAHB left anterior hemiblock
LATS long-acting thyroid stimulator
LAV lymphadenopathy-associated virus
LBBB left bundle branch block
LCF left circumflex (coronary artery)
LCX left circumflex (coronary artery)
LDH lactic dehydrogenase
LDL low-density lipoprotein
LE prep lupus erythematosus preparation
LFT latex flocculation test
   left frontotransverse
   liver function tests
LGA large for gestational age
LGL Lown-Ganong-Levine (syndrome)
LICM left intercostal margin
LICS left intercostal space
LIH left inguinal hernia
LIMA left internal mammary artery
LLE left lower extremity
LLL left lower lid
LLQ left lower quadrant (abdomen)
LM left main (coronary artery)
LMCA left main coronary artery
LMP last menstrual period
   left mentoposterior
LOA leave of absence
   left occiput anterior
   looseness of associations
   lysis of adhesions
LOP left occiput posterior
LOS length of stay
LOT left occiput transverse
LOV loss of vision
LPFB left posterior fascicular block
LPH left posterior hemiblock
LSA left sacrum anterior
   lymphosarcoma
LSC late systolic click
   lichen simplex chronicus
LSM late systolic murmur
LSTL laparoscopic tubal ligation
LTL laparoscopic tubal ligation
LUL left upper lid
   left upper lobe (lung)
LUQ left upper quadrant (abdoman)
LV left ventricle
LVAD left ventricular assist device

LVAT left ventricular activation time
LVD left ventricular dysfunction
LVDP left ventricular diastolic pressure
LVDV left ventricular diastolic volume
LVE left ventricular enlargement
LVEDP left ventricular end-diastolic pressure
LVEDV left ventricular end-diastolic volume
LVEF left ventricular ejection fraction
LVET left ventricular ejection time
LVF left ventricular failure
LVFP left ventricular filling pressure
LVH left ventricular hypertrophy
LVOT left ventricular outflow tract

M

MAHA microangiopathic hemolytic anemia
MAST mastectomy
MB-CK isozyme of creatine kinase
MCH mean corpuscular hemoglobin
MCHC mean corpuscular hemoglobin concentration
MCL medial collateral ligament
   midclavicular line
   modified chest lead
MCTD mixed connective tissue disease
MCV mean corpuscular volume
MEA-I multiple endocrine adenomatosis, type I
MEFV maximum expiratory flow volume
mEq milliequivalent
META metamyelocytes
MM malignant melanoma
   Marshall-Marchetti
   medial malleolus
   millimeter
   multiple myeloma
MMR measles, mumps, and rubella
MMS Mini-Mental State (examination)
MODM maturity onset diabetes mellitus
MOPP mechlorethamine, vincristine, procarbazine, and prednisone
MOPV monovalent oral poliovirus vaccine
MRM modified radical mastectomy
MRSA methicillin-resistant *Staphylococcus aureus*
MRSE methicillin-resistant *Staphylococcus epidermidis*
MSAP mean systemic arterial pressure
MSL midsternal line
MSM midsystolic murmur

MTX methotrexate
MVO mixed venous oxygen saturation
MVO$_2$ myocardial oxygen consumption
MYR myringotomy

N

NABS normoactive bowel sound
NANB non-A, non-B (hepatitis)
NANBH non-A, non-B hepatitis
NC/AT normocephalic atraumatic (cranium)
NCB natural childbirth
NCNC normochromic, normocytic
NDI neurogenic diabetes insipidus
NEM no evidence of malignancy
NFTD normal full-term delivery
NFTSD normal full-term spontaneous delivery
NIAL not in active labor
NID not in distress
NIDD non-insulin-dependent diabetes
NIDDM non-insulin-dependent diabetes mellitus
NIL not in labor
NKC nonketotic coma
NKHA nonketotic hypersomolar acidosis
NKHS nonketotic hypersomolar syndrome
NKMA no known medication allergies
NLP no light perception
NLS neonatal lupus syndrome
NMP normal menstrual period
NMR nuclear magnetic resonance (magnetic resonance imaging)
NOK next of kin
NPH isophane insulin
NQMI non-Q wave myocardial infarction
NRF normal renal function
NSAD no signs of acute disease
NSAIA nonsteroidal anti-inflammatory agent
NSAID nonsteroidal anti-inflammatory drug
NSBGP nonspecific bowel gas pattern
NSHD nodular sclerosing Hodgkin's disease
NSR normal sinus rhythm
NSSTT nonspecific ST and T (wave)
NSU neurosurgical unit
nonspecific urethritis
NSV nonspecific vaginitis
NSVD normal spontaneous vaginal delivery
NSVT nonsustained ventricular tachycardia
NTG nitroglycerin
N & V nausea and vomiting

NVDC nausea, vomiting, diarrhea, and constipation
NYHA New York Heart Association (heart disease classification)

O

OD once daily (**bad abbreviation**)
optic disc
overdose
right eye
OKN optokinetic nystagmus
OOB out of bed
OOL onset of labor
OOP out of pelvis
OPD outpatient department
OS left eye
occipitosacral
opening snap
oral surgery
OSAS obstructive sleep apnea syndrome
OU both eyes

P

P & A percussion and auscultation
P$_2$ > A$_2$ pulmonic second heart sound is greater than the aortic second heart sound
PAGA premature appropriate for gestational age
PAP primary atypical pneumonia
prostatic acid phosphatase
Pap smear Papanicolaou smear
PARA number of pregnancies
PAT paroxysmal atrial tachycardia
PCG phonocardiogram
PCH paroxysmal cold hemoglobinurea
PCKD polycystic kidney disease
PCN penicillin
PCO polycystic ovary
PCOS polycystic ovarian syndrome
PCP *Pneumocystis carinii* pneumonia
pulmonary capillary pressure
PDA patent ductus arteriosus
posterior descending (coronary) artery
PE physical examination
pulmonary edema
pulmonary embolism
PEARL pupils equal accommodation, reactive to light
PEEP positive end-expiratory pressure
PEG pneumoencephalogram

PERRLA pupils equal, round, and reactive to light and accommodation
PGA prostaglandin A
PGE₁ prostaglandin E_1 (alprostadil)
PGE₂ prostaglandin E_2 (dinoprostone)
PGI potassium, glucose, and insulin
PGY postgraduate year
Ph¹ Philadelphia chromosome
PHACO phacoemulsification
PHR peak heart rate
PHx past (medical) history
PIF peak inspiratory flow
PKD polycystic kidney disease
PLR pupillary light reflex
PMH past medical history
PMN polymorphonuclear leukocyte
PND paroxysmal nocturnal dyspnea
   pelvic node dissection
   postnasal drip
   pregnancy-not delivered
PNH paroxysmal nocturnal hemoglobinurea
PO *per os* (by mouth)
   postoperative
POL premature onset of labor
POMP prednisone, vincristine, methotrexate and mercaptopurine
PP & A palpation, percussion, and auscultation
PPD packs per day
   postpartum day
   purified protein derivative (tuberculin test)
PPH postpartum hemorrhage
   primary pulmonary hypertension
PRD polycystic renal disease
P/S polyunsaturated to saturated fatty acid ratio
PSA prostatic-specific antigen
PSVT paroxysmal supraventricular tachycardia
PTHC percutaneous transhepatic cholangiography
PTT partial thromboplastin time
   platelet transfusion therapy
PUA pelvic (examination) under anesthesia
PVC polyvinyl chloride
   postvoiding cystogram
   premature ventricular contraction
   pulmonary venous congestion
PVR peripheral vascular resistance
   postvoiding residual

   proliferative vitreoretinopathy
   pulmonary vascular resistance
PVT paroxysmal ventricular tachycardia
PXE pseudoxanthoma elasticum

Q

q every
QA quality assurance
qd daily (**DO NOT USE**—may be mistaken for 4 times a day)
q4h every 4 hours
qhs at bedtime
qid four times a day
qod alternate days (**DO NOT USE**—may be mistaken for 4 times a day or every day)
QOL quality of life

R

RAE right atrial enlargement
RAP right atrial pressure
RCV red cell volume
RDOD retinal detachment—right eye
RDOS retinal detachment—left eye
retic reticulocyte
Rh Rhesus factor (blood)
RhoGAM $Rh_0(D)$ immune globulin
RIA radioimmunoassay
RICM right intercostal margin
RICS right intercostal space
RIH right inguinal hernia
RK radial keratotomy
RLE right lower extremity
RLL right lower lid
   right lower lobe
RLQ right lower quadrant (abdomen)
RML right middle lobe
R/O rule out
ROA right occiput anterior
ROM range of motion
   right otitis media
ROP right occiput posterior
ROS review of systems
RSA right sacrum anterior
   right subclavian artery
RTC return to clinic
RUL right upper lobe
RUQ right upper quadrant (abdome0n)
RVH right ventricular hypertrophy
RVO right ventricular outflow (tract)

RVOT right ventricular outflow tract
RVP right ventricular pressure
RVT renal vein thrombosis

S

S$_1$ first heart sound
sacral vertebra 1
S$_2$ second heart sound
sacral vertebra 2
S$_3$ third heart sound (ventricular gallop)
sacral vertebra 3
S$_4$ fourth heart sound (atrial gallop)
sacral vertebra 4
SCC small cell carcinoma
SDH subdural hematoma
SEM scanning electronic microscope
SGA small for gestational age
SGOT serum glutamic oxaloacetic transaminase (AST)
SGPT serum glutamic pyruvic transaminase (ALT)
SIADH syndrome of inappropriate antidiuretic hormone
SICU surgical intensive care unit
SLE slit-lamp examination
systemic lupus erythematosus
SMA-6 sequential multiplier analyzer (sodium, potassium, CO_2, chloride, glucose, and blood urea nitrogen)
SMA-12 sequential multiplier analyzer (glucose, blood urea nitrogen, uric acid, calcium, phosphorus, total protein albumin, cholesterol, total bilirubin, alkaline phosphatase, SGOT, and LDH)
SO suboccipital
superior oblique
supraoptic
sutures out
SOAP subjective, objective, assessment, and plan
SOB shortness of breath
SPEP serum protein electrophoresis
SROM spontaneous rupture of membrane
SSD sickle cell disease
STD sexually transmitted disease
STIs systolic time intervals

T

T$_3$ triiodothyroxine

thoracic vertebra 3
thoracic nerve 3
T$_4$ levothyroxine
thyroxine
thoracic vertebra 4
thoracic nerve 4
T & A tonsillectomy and adenoidectomy
TAH total abdominal hysterectomy
TAPVD total anomalous pulmonary venous drainage
TBB transbronchial biopsy
TBG thyroxine-binding globulin
TBLB transbronchial lung biopsy
Tc technetium
TDN transdermal nitroglycerin
TDNTG transdermal nitroglycerin
TEE transesophageal echocardiography
TENS transcutaneous electrical nerve stimulation
TEP tracheoesophageal puncture
TEV *talipes equinovarus* (club foot deformity)
TFTs thyroid function tests
TG triglycerides
TGA transposition of the great arteries
TIA transient ischemic attack
TIBC total iron binding capacity
TID three times a day
TIUP term intrauterine pregnancy
TKO to keep open
TLE temporal lobe epilepsy
T & M type and crossmatch
TNBP transurethral needle biopsy of the prostate
TNG nitroglycerin
TOA tubo-ovarian abscess
TOP termination of pregnancy
TOT BILI total bilirubin
TPA tissue plasminogen activator
TRIG triglycerides
TSE testicular self-examination
TSH thyroid-stimulating hormone
TTE transthoracic echocardiography
TTNA transthoracic needle aspiration
TTP thrombotic thrombocytopenic purpura
TUIP transurethral incision of the prostate
TULIP transurethral ultrasound-guided laser-induced prostatectomy
TUPR transurethral prostatic resection
TUR transurethral resection
TURP transurethral resection of the prostate

TVF tactile vocal fremitus
TVH total vaginal hysterectomy
TWE tapwater enema
TWETC tapwater enema till clear

U

UA urinalysis
UCG urnary chorionic gonadotropins
UCX urine culture
UES upper esophageal sphincter
UGI upper gastrointestinal (series)
UPEP urine protein electrophoresis
UPJ ureteropelvic junction
UROB urobilinogen
USG ultrasonography
USOGH usual state of good health
USOH usual state of health
UTD up-to-date

V

VAGHYST vaginal hysterectomy
VAOD visual acuity—right eye
VAOS visual acuity—left eye
VBAC vaginal birth after cesarean
VCU voiding cystourethrogram
V & D vomiting and diarrhea
VLDL very low density lipoprotein
VOD veno-occlusive disease
VPB ventricular premature beat
VPC ventricular premature contraction
VSN vital signs normal
VT ventricular tachycardia
v. tach. ventricular tachycardia
VV varicose veins
VWD von Willebrand's disease
vWF von Willebrand's factor

W

WAP wandering atrial pacemaker
WD well developed
WDHA watery diarrhea, hypokalemia, and achlorhydria
WDLL well-differentiated lymphocytic leukemia
WHO World Health Organization
WKD Wernicke-Korsakoff syndrome
WN well nourished
WNL within normal limits

WRBC washed red blood cells

X

X3 orientation as to time, place, and person
XM crossmatch
XX normal female sex chromosome type
XY normal male sex chromosome type
XYL Xylocaine
XYLO Xylocaine

Y

YAG yttrium aluminum garnet (laser)
YO year old

Z

Z-E Zollinger-Ellison (syndrome)
ZES Zollinger-Ellison syndrome

SYMBOLS

↑ elevated
  high
  increase
  rising

↓ depressed
  low
  decrease
  falling

→ results in
  showed

↓↓ testes descended

∴ therefore

+ plus
  positive
  present

− minus
  negative
  absent

± plus or minus
  very slight trace

> greater than

≥ greater than or equal to

< less than

≤ less than or equal to

≈ approximately
? questionable

@ at
1° first degree
  primary
2° second degree
  secondary
3° third degree
  tertiary

♂ male

♀ female

■ deceased male

● deceased female

□ living male

○ living female

† dead

Index

Note: Page numbers in *italics* refer to illustrations; page numbers followed by t refer to tables.

261